CLINICAL GUIDELINE DEVELOPMENT

AN ALGORITHM APPROACH

James P. Mozena, MST
President
The Mozena Consulting Group
Troutdale, Oregon

Charles E. Emerick, MS, ATC
Clinic Manager
Providence Centralia Physical Therapy
Centralia, Washington

Steven C. Black, MPT, PT
Director
Providence Physical Therapy
Centralia, Washington

Consulting Physician

Carl R. Birchard, MD, AAOS, ABOS
Orthopaedic Surgeon
Washington Orthopaedic Center
Centralia, Washington

AN ASPEN PUBLICATION©

Aspen Publishers, Inc.
Gaithersburg, Maryland
1996

Library of Congress Cataloging-in-Publication Data

Mozena, James P., 1949–
Clinical guideline development : an algorithm approach / James P.
Mozena, Charles E. Emerick, Steven C. Black.
p. cm.
Includes bibliographical references and index.
ISBN 0-8342-0734-6
1. Medical protocols. I. Emerick, Charles E. II. Black, Steven C.
III. Title.
[DNLM: 1. Practice Guidelines. 2. Algorithms. 3. Physical
Therapy—standards. W 84.1 M939c 1996]
RC64.M69 1996
362.1'068'5—dc20
DNLM/DLC
for Library of Congress
95-39261
CIP

Copyright © 1996 by Aspen Publishers, Inc.

Aspen Publishers, Inc., grants permission for photocopying for limited personal or internal use. This consent does not extend to other kinds of copying, such as copying for general distribution, for advertising or promotional purposes, for creating new collective works, or for resale. For information, address Aspen Publishers, Inc., Permissions Department, 200 Orchard Ridge Drive, Suite 200, Gaithersburg, Maryland 20878.

Editorial Resources: Ruth Bloom

Library of Congress Catalog Card Number: 95-39261
ISBN: 0-8342-0734-6

Printed in the United States of America

1   2   3   4   5

_____

_____

*This book is dedicated to all the associates of Black Hills
Physical Therapy. The successful completion of this project
would not have been possible without their support, guidance,
and friendship. Special recognition is also given to Providence
Centralia Hospital and Washington Orthopaedic Center for
their many years of support and direction.*

_____

_____

Table of Contents

Foreword

The health professions are learning professions. Every clinician, as a condition to entry into the caring services, agrees to observe the treatments they offer to their patients and the outcomes they achieve, with an aim to improve their treatments for future patients. Among physicians, for example, that core ideal defines the "practice" of medicine. It is the foundation upon which the medical profession rests. Physicians embrace that essential value as part of their medical school and residency training experience. In different forms the other health professions claim the same touchstone. All health professionals commit to continue to learn throughout their careers, as part of their fundamental commitment to their patients.

Clinicians learn another core concept during their professional training: you can't trust subjective data. In one very real sense, the practice of medicine—in fact, the practice of any of the health professions—is an information science. The better data you have, the better diagnosis you can achieve on behalf of your patients. For that reason, much of clinical training revolves around the capture and synthesis of *objective* information. A broad body of research has repeatedly demonstrated that human beings are notoriously poor at summarizing information subjectively, especially across groups of patients or over time.

Taken together these two core values give rise to critical questions for health professionals: How do we learn from our own clinical experience? How can we gain objective, *valid* clinical knowledge as we serve those who come to us for help, so that we are better able to serve others in the future? What methods will better let us learn from the clinical experience of our colleagues, not just through published scientific studies, but from patients treated by other health professionals in our clinics, in our hospitals, or in our community?

The fact is that every clinician uses clinical algorithms to accomplish the daily work of caring for patients. When I was a medical student and intern, I carried my algorithms around in the pocket of my lab coat, in the form of a *Washington Manual*. Eventually I moved those algorithms—modified by knowledge that I gained from my instructors, from lectures, from journal articles, and from other sources— out of my pocket and into my head. But still, to this day, for every patient I see, I start with my standard diagnostic protocol; then, having made a diagnosis, I move on to my standard therapeutic protocol for the particular condition I believe my patient displays. I do not use my protocols uncritically; I know that I will need to customize my standard approach to meet the specific, unique needs of each patient I encounter. Every physician—every clinician—follows the same pattern when they care for patients. But to actually be the continually learning and growing health professionals that we hope to be, our internal protocols suffer from two grievous diseases of our own: They rely upon our subjective judgment as we assess the treatments we apply and the outcomes we achieve subjectively, in our heads; and they exclude the patient care experiences of our colleagues.

Formal clinical algorithms address both of these deficiencies. By moving my internal protocols from my head to a sheet of paper, they make it possible to understand, to criticize, to share, and to improve. I can learn not just from my own thoughts and experiences, but from my colleagues' insights and experiences. If I share a standard approach to a particular clinical problem with my colleagues, it increases my sample size. I gain better, more objective, more valid treatment and outcome information not just from my patients but from those similar patients treated in similar ways by my associates. The algorithm also gives me a framework within which to interpret my clinical experience. A written clinical algorithm, backed up by an objective tracking system and applied across a group of collaborating clinicians, improves the quality and quantity of information I have available to learn from my clinical experience. In the extreme, an algorithm designed to support daily clinical practice can serve as the control arm of a formal randomized controlled clinical trial, the gold standard in our professional search for valid new treatment knowledge. In my own institution and in other health care delivery organizations around the United States and Canada, clinical groups are presently using treatment algorithms in exactly that manner.

As the authors of this textbook correctly point out, most health care delivery organizations plan to use clinical algorithms for case management. They can justify the effort of developing, implementing, and tracking treatment protocols solely on the basis of the cost savings that these tools often produce. But the importance of clinical algorithms extends far beyond that mundane (if legitimate) need: Clinical algorithms offer a singular opportunity to bring together groups of clinicians to achieve the core values upon which the health professions are built. They provide a better framework by which we can "practice" health care. They are a critical element to help us understand the treatments we give to our patients, and the outcomes we achieve, so that in the future we can deliver better treatments and outcomes to the patients who depend upon us.

Brent C. James, MD, MStat
Vice President for Medical Research
Executive Director
Institute for Health Care Delivery Research
Intermountain Health Care
Salt Lake City, Utah

Preface

Medicine in the 1990s is under assault by threats and pressures from government agencies, third-party payers, businesses, and consumers. The pressures are even coming from entities that seem to have no names—only initials—such as DRGs, RVRBS, HEDIS, RVUs, and HCFA. All of these are challenging the clinician to quantify, standardize, and improve the cost-effectiveness of clinical activities.

In response to these challenges, clinicians have become familiar with a wide variety of clinical improvement methods. These include, but are not limited to, critical care pathways, clinical outcome studies, evidence-based medicine, physician profiling, protocol development, care paths, clinical maps, and clinical pathways. These methods belong to a growing field, known as clinical guideline development.

In this volume, we are presenting a structured, step-by-step approach that facilitates improvements within any organization. Even though the use of the word *algorithm* may be confusing to some, the structure itself is merely a graphic representation of a clinical guideline. The algorithm uses the fundamental scientific approach to clinical improvement and presents a sequential progression of the logic needed for effective clinical decision making.

Our attempts at developing clinical algorithms began approximately five years ago. At that time, we recognized that we needed to standardize our clinical processes before we could truly understand them and improve upon them. We also quickly learned that the creation and implementation of a clinical algorithm are difficult processes that involve many stages.

Because an algorithm is complex, we conducted literature searches for information on how actually to create and implement an algorithm. Although many publications discussed the advantages and merits of using clinical algorithms, none gave us the "how-to" knowledge of proceeding from conception to implementation.

Through our experiences, attendance at educational events, and consultations with experts in the field of clinical improvement, we have developed this handbook to provide a practical, step-by-step approach so that health care providers can develop and use algorithms in their clinical practice. We believe that any clinician who wants to understand and improve upon his or her clinical outcomes will benefit by following this approach.

Introduction

The algorithm, or the step-by-step approach to solving problems, was the brainchild of the Persian mathematician Al-khaforizmi, who invented it in the ninth century. The technique's original purpose was to solve arithmetic problems. The advent of the computer in the middle of the twentieth century mandated the rapid development of such step-by-step solutions. Experts had to develop logical methods of instruction to enable operators to direct a computer effectively.

For the past 25 years, this same type of approach has been slowly making headway into the field of medicine. Medical authors began in the late 1960s to discuss the use of such a stepwise approach to solving the problems faced in the everyday clinical setting.[1,2] This is an environment ideally suited to the use of algorithms, as clinicians must make a series of sequential decisions in caring for each patient to determine the appropriate treatment for that patient. A fully developed algorithm can facilitate this decision-making process and help ensure that the patient receives optimum care.

Certainly, guidelines in medicine are not new. Every medical textbook describes the approximate course of treatment, given a certain set of symptoms. As far back as the times described in the Old Testament, medical guidelines were common. The book of Leviticus, for example, contains a discussion of the symptoms and treatment of leprosy; it includes instructions that advised the priests of the day to look at the hair and the skin of those who may be afflicted with leprosy. Based on their findings, they were then instructed to treat the patient in a certain manner. Thus, the priests used a primitive form of an algorithm during the decision-making process regarding such a patient.

Although such guidelines have been part of medicine for more than 3,000 years, the medical community has been reluctant to embrace the detailed, step-by-step approach that an algorithm provides. One of the earliest proponents of algorithms, Margolis, noted three common objections to the use of clinical algorithms in medicine.[3]

First, the most often given objection is that algorithms will turn physicians into robots who do not have to think. Every medical discipline has critics of the "cookbook" approach for treating patients. According to these critics, physicians who use algorithms will gather information from the patient and simply turn to the relevant box in the algorithm to determine the appropriate treatment. The critics contend that this approach will hold any thinking on the part of the physician to a minimum. Margolis argued just the opposite, however. In his view, the use of a structured approach to clinical problem solving actually facilitates thinking about a clinical problem, because it enables the practitioner to think more clearly about the situation. Furthermore, an algorithm is especially useful for medical situations that the clinician does not regularly encounter. It provides a framework for the decision-making process since it assists the practitioner by providing a logical sequence of considerations used by other clinicians who are considered experts in the field.

Second, the critics commonly object to clinical algorithms on the ground that they are general and will not be applicable to a specific patient. Margolis agreed that every patient is unique. Only after a careful and thorough examination by the physician will a patient fit into an algorithm. At every decision-making point along the way, the clinician decides if this unique patient fits into the algorithm.

Finally, as Margolis noted, some authorities believe that not all physicians are able to think "algorithmically." Experienced clinicians acknowledge that they follow an algorithm in their head whenever examining a patient, however. Thus, although an algorithm written into an official document may be somewhat intimidating, it represents a technique that experienced clinicians actually use on a daily basis.

The persuasive arguments of Margolis notwithstanding, many clinicians continue to express concern over the use of algorithms in medicine. They perceive algorithms as restrictive and fear that algorithms will limit the clinician in practicing the "art" of medicine. Because of these objections, the use of algorithms in medicine has had a dismal record. It has been very difficult to get clinicians to accept algorithms. As a result, very few have been successfully implemented.

In the current environment of health care reform, ever increasing numbers of consumers, legislators, insurance companies, government agencies, businesses, and professional health care organizations are demanding affordable, appropriate health care. It is essential to stabilize and standardize clinical processes so that all these health care consumers can understand, manage, contain, and compare the costs of various treatments.

Not only are these entities demanding efficient use of financial resources, but also they are demanding health care decisions that are based on the clinically accepted "best practice" for a medical situation. By definition, a clinical algorithm is exactly that. It is a problem-solving approach that is based on scientific evidence regarding a clinical activity or situation; in other words, an algorithm exemplifies "best practice."

The term *best practice* appears often in this handbook. It is the reason that algorithms are used and used effectively. Best practice has three components:

1. optimal clinical outcome
2. optimal cost efficiency
3. optimal service attributes

While the first two components are easily understood, the third—optimal service attributes—is not. The term indicates a clinical process so efficient and optimal that every interaction with that patient is a positive experience. The interaction will also be positive for the clinician who understands the importance of meeting the needs of the patient. Knowing that the patient is receiving the best care available within the organization, the clinician gets satisfaction, too. Leaving the office, the patient has the feeling that the medical organization has met or exceeded each of his or her needs. An effective clinical algorithm takes all three components into account in defining best practice for a particular organization.

Furthermore, when successful, a clinical algorithm stabilizes and standardizes clinical processes within a particular diagnosis. As scientists, all clinicians understand that only after clinical processes have been stabilized is it possible to understand and methodically predict clinical outcomes. If the results of an experiment (or treatment activity) are to be valid and reliable, processes must be stabilized and variables controlled as much as possible. An algorithm provides the scientific basis for such stabilization.

Another positive result of the use of clinical algorithms is that they allow clinicians to analyze the time spent on each activity.[4] Like most of life, the practice of medicine is governed by the Pareto (or 80/20) Rule. This rule states that 80 percent of clinical outcomes are achieved by 20 percent of clinical activities. The algorithm makes it possible to analyze actions, eliminate inefficiencies, and optimize the resources of both the clinician and the patient. The ability to focus on a few vital steps in a clinical process enables clinicians to become more efficient, and therefore, they can decrease patient costs, increase revenue for the organization, and increase their satisfaction.

Thus, by creating and using clinical algorithms, clinicians can ensure that they are providing their patients with the care accepted as best practice. The clinical outcome is optimal for the patient, both the provider and the patient effectively use their resources, and the provider receives the ancillary benefits of providing quality service to the community at large.

The remaining chapters of this handbook provide a structured, step-by-step approach on the development and implementation of algorithms in a health care organization. This text is designed to be used as a workbook for the algorithm team members. It contains a discussion of each step of the algorithm process. After each of these, there are forms for the team members to review and complete. Although most are self-explanatory, additional information and some "helpful hints" facilitate the completion of the step. As the team members successfully complete the forms, their understanding of the algorithm process will greatly increase, and the algorithm will have a much greater chance of success within the organization. At the end of the process, clinicians will have agreed on best practice, clinical processes for a particular diagnosis will have been standardized, and resources of both the patient and clinician will have been optimized. In the current climate of health care reform, any one of these results is reason enough to use clinical algorithms.

NOTES

1. B.N. Lewis and G. Pask, *Case Studies in the Use of Algorithms* (London: Pergamon Press, 1967).
2. L. Lusted, *An Introduction to Medical Decision Making* (Springfield, IL: Charles C. Thomas, 1968).
3. C.Z. Margolis, Uses of Clinical Algorithms, *JAMA* 249 (1983):627–632.
4. P.R. Scholtes, *The Team Handbook* (Madison, WI: Joiner Associates, 1987).

ALGORITHM FLOWCHART

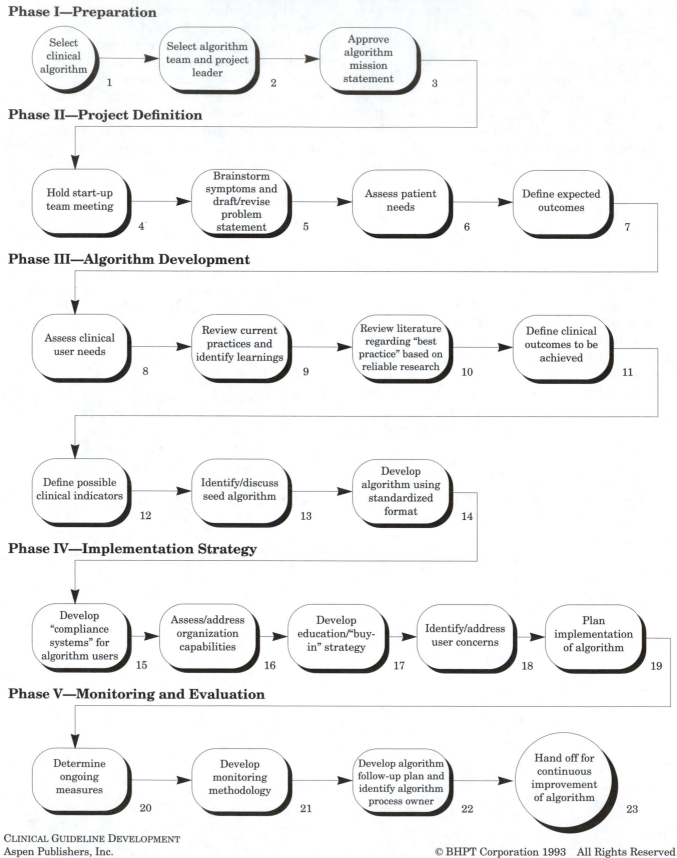

Phase I—Preparation

Select clinical algorithm `1` → Select algorithm team and project leader `2` → Approve algorithm mission statement `3`

Phase II—Project Definition

Hold start-up team meeting `4` → Brainstorm symptoms and draft/revise problem statement `5` → Assess patient needs `6` → Define expected outcomes `7`

Phase III—Algorithm Development

Assess clinical user needs `8` → Review current practices and identify learnings `9` → Review literature regarding "best practice" based on reliable research `10` → Define clinical outcomes to be achieved `11`

Define possible clinical indicators `12` → Identify/discuss seed algorithm `13` → Develop algorithm using standardized format `14`

Phase IV—Implementation Strategy

Develop "compliance systems" for algorithm users `15` → Assess/address organization capabilities `16` → Develop education/"buy-in" strategy `17` → Identify/address user concerns `18` → Plan implementation of algorithm `19`

Phase V—Monitoring and Evaluation

Determine ongoing measures `20` → Develop monitoring methodology `21` → Develop algorithm follow-up plan and identify algorithm process owner `22` → Hand off for continuous improvement of algorithm `23`

CLINICAL GUIDELINE DEVELOPMENT
Aspen Publishers, Inc.

Phase I

○ ○ ○ ○

Preparation: Beginning the Project

As long as practitioners have been treating patients and recording the results, they have been developing clinical guidelines. From century-old textbooks to the most recent article in the medical journals, guidelines for appropriate care are continually being presented.

Practitioners—either consciously or subconsciously—follow various types of guidelines in their treatment of patients. They may rely on a detailed algorithm, a familiar protocol, or a little book that they carry in their lab coat pocket. With any of these tools, practitioners are using guidelines to help them choose the best treatment for their patients.

As can be imagined, the use of many clinical decision-making tools can result in a wide variation between the treatment plans of two practitioners in the same state, the same city, or even the same building. This handbook represents an opportunity for practitioners to eliminate this variation and to define best practice for their patients.

Three elements are involved in an organization's clinical algorithm development effort:

1. a senior quality council
2. an algorithm steering group
3. the algorithm team

The first of these, the senior quality council, is made up of senior level clinicians, administrators, and executives within the organization. This council has the ultimate responsibility for the quality of medical care within the clinic/hospital/organization. In the algorithm effort, the senior quality council has four specific responsibilities:

1. selection and/or approval of the members of the algorithm steering group
2. final approval of a major algorithm development effort so that the algorithm is consistent with the goals and strategies of the organization
3. evaluation of the overall effectiveness of the algorithm development effort
4. resolution of political, structural, or financial barriers within the organization that would inhibit the successful implementation of the algorithm

An organization desiring to begin the algorithm process should designate an algorithm steering group to ensure that the algorithm team follows the framework of the four-phase algorithm development flowchart. Depending on the size of the organization, this group usually consists of four or five people who are medical quality managers, senior practitioners, chiefs of the various staffs, and/or senior medical office administrators. In general, the role of the algorithm steering group is to guide and support the algorithm team throughout the development process; they are responsible for the overall management of this algorithm development effort. The specific duties of the steering group include:

- selecting the clinical process to be studied.

- selecting the members of the algorithm team. The steering group must ensure that all the appropriate disciplines are represented on the algorithm team.
- securing the resources necessary for the algorithm team to perform its work.
- developing a mission statement for the project. This includes a problem statement, expected outcomes, key indicators, expectations, and constraints.
- approving the final mission statement after the algorithm team has revised it.

Step 1

○ ○ ○ ○ ○

Select Clinical Algorithm

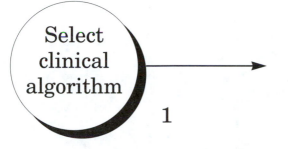

Of the steering group's duties, the most important one is the selection of the clinical process to be examined. Members of the steering group must consider the following questions in choosing an algorithm that will have the greatest positive impact on the existing practice:

- Once the algorithm has been completed, how difficult will its implementation be?
- What is the potential financial cost of implementation?
- How often during the day is this treatment activity occurring?
- Does this treatment activity take up a great deal of time during an average day?
- Will the algorithm have a high return for the resources needed to develop it?
- Does this process (or treatment activity) have a high impact on patient satisfaction?
- Is this treatment activity the most frustrating for the clinicians?
- Does this activity give the clinicians the least satisfactory results?
- Will the algorithm address current goals/issues facing the medical practice or organization?
- Will the clinicians be willing to use ("buy into") the completed algorithm?

NOTES

A form should be developed so that each member of the steering group can use questions such as these to evaluate potential algorithms. (See Resources 1–1 and 1–2 on algorithm selection criteria.) After compiling the data from these forms, the steering group decides if a potential algorithm is appropriate.

Once a topic gains approval, the steering group drafts the initial version of the mission statement. (For information on developing a mission statement and for a sample, see Resources 1–3 through 1–5.) The steering group then turns its attention to the selection of the algorithm team.

NOTES

Resource 1–1

○ ○ ○ ○ ○

Algorithm Selection

There are several methods by which the steering group may become aware of clinical processes that should be studied. The most common of these methods are medical quality assurance/management activities, peer reviews, utilization studies, requests from group purchasers regarding utilization and/or cost information, results from group purchasers regarding utilization and/or cost information, results of reviews of regulatory agencies (e.g., Joint Commission on Accreditation of Healthcare Organizations), and comments of concerned clinicians.

From the countless clinical diagnostic/treatment activities that occur throughout the day, the steering group chooses one for assignment to an algorithm team. To assist the steering group in this task, a form such as that shown in Resource 1–2 provides an objective way to assess the cost:benefit potential of initiating an algorithm development project.

Members of the algorithm steering group can complete such a form within the meeting or prior to the meeting. Like any survey, however, it only provides indicators of the importance of the potential algorithm. The steering group needs to discuss the results of the survey thoroughly and reach consensus on the clinical activity that is selected for improvement.

HELPFUL HINTS

- The definition of consensus is that all members of the steering group can "live with" the decision. When members leave the meeting, they must be willing to support the group decision in discussions with their peers and stakeholders of the clinical activity to be examined.

- The steering group may consider sending the results of the survey to the clinicians who will be most affected by any changes caused by the new algorithm. This may be the first step in gaining a "buy-in" by those who will be actually using the algorithm on a daily basis.

Resource 1–2

○ ○ ○ ○ ○

Algorithm Selection: Criteria

_____   _____
Algorithm Title   **Date**

As a member of the algorithm steering group, please evaluate the following treatment activity for determination if an algorithm effort is appropriate. Please answer each question with a number rating of 1 through 7.

_____
(Treatment Activity)

____ 1. To what extent will this algorithm improve clinical practice of this treatment activity (1, greatly improve–7, slightly improve)

____ 2. To what extent will the completed algorithm be difficult to implement? (1, not difficult–7, very difficult)

____ 3. What is the potential financial cost of implementing this algorithm? (1, minimal–7, significant)

____ 4. How often during the day does this treatment activity occur? (1, very often–7, rarely)

____ 5. How much time does this clinical activity take up during an average day? (1, great deal–7, virtually none)

____ 6. To what extent will the algorithm have a high return for the resources needed to develop it? (1, high return–7, low return)

____ 7. To what extent will this algorithm have an impact on patient satisfaction (1, high impact–7, low impact)

____ 8. To what extent is this treatment activity frustrating for the clinicians (1, very frustrating–7, slightly frustrating)

____ 9. To what extent does this treatment activity produce unsatisfactory results? (1, often–7, rarely)

____ 10. To what extent will this algorithm address current goals/issues facing the organization? (1, does address–7, does not address)

____ 11. To what extent will the clinicians be willing to use ("buy into") the completed algorithm? (1, very likely–7, unlikely)

Additional comments concerning this potential algorithm:

_____

_____

_____

Resource 1–3

○ ○ ○ ○ ○

Mission Statement
for Algorithm Project

The first draft of the mission statement for the algorithm project is the responsibility of the algorithm steering group. To prepare this draft, the steering group should first gather all the information that triggered the request for the algorithm. The steering group may ask other departments within the organization (e.g., quality management, financial planning, medical economics, management engineering) to collect data as well to increase the validity of the algorithm.

The steering group uses these data to clarify the scope of the algorithm development effort. In other words, the steering group decides what will be included and excluded during the deliberations of the algorithm team. Furthermore, the steering group determines how the potential effects of the algorithm will be measured.

It may not be as easy as it seems to develop an effective mission statement. There must be a balance between generality and detail. A mission statement that is too general may not provide the team with enough clarity to focus the limited time and resources expeditiously. One that is too detailed may bias the team's objectivity and jeopardize the validity of the entire project.

HELPFUL HINTS

- Using the information that was previously obtained, the group should be able to draft the initial mission statement in one meeting.

- The team must "own" the algorithm development effort; thus, the team must develop a thorough understanding of the symptoms related to the clinical activity to be reviewed. To ensure that these goals are accomplished, the team draws on the experience of the team members and clinicians who actually "live within" the clinical system being studied for the mission statement.

- A mission statement differs from a problem statement. The mission statement describes the overall scope of the project, which includes such items as the problem statement, expected outcomes, and possible measures. The problem statement, included in the mission statement, objectively describes the current situation. It describes the impact of the situation without offering a solution or placing blame.

- A sample mission statement is provided as Resource 1–5.

Resource 1–4

○ ○ ○ ○ ○

Mission Statement for Algorithm Project: Suggested Format

_____   _____
Algorithm Title   **Date**

    Problem Statement: _____

    _____

    _____

    _____

    Expected Outcomes: _____

    _____

    _____

    _____

    Possible Key Indicators: _____

    _____

    _____

    _____

    Expectations: _____

    _____

    _____

    _____

    Constraints: _____

    _____

    _____

    _____

    Algorithm Team Members: _____

    _____

    _____

    _____

    Desired Project Completion Date:_____

Resource 1–5

○ ○ ○ ○ ○

Mission Statement for Algorithm Project: Sample

Date: 13 October 1996

Project Title: Utilization Rates for Management of Patients with Angina

Problem Statement: Within our health maintenance organization, the utilization rates for management of patients with angina vary greatly.

Expected Outcomes:

1. Identify causes for differences in utilization rates.
2. Develop consensus of best practice regarding management of patients with the diagnosis of angina.
3. Develop an algorithm and educational program for the physicians involved with the treatment of patients with angina.

Key Indicators:

1. Length of hospital stay for patients with angina
2. Physician visits for patients with angina

Expectations:

1. Algorithm will be developed with input from the department of cardiology.
2. A report will be made to the steering group at the end of Phase I.
3. Benchmarking will be done with health maintenance organizations of similar size throughout the United States.

Constraints:

1. Diagnosis other than angina must be approved by the steering group before being considered by the team.
2. Significant cost recommendations must be analyzed by the financial planning department.

Algorithm Team Members:

Ralph King, MD, Internal Medicine, Project Leader
Mona Prankus, MD, Internal Medicine
Chuck Smoker, MD, Cardiology
Martin Egolf, MD, Emergency
Linda Higgens, RN, Emergency
Sheila Hopkins, MS, Director of Cardiac Services
Mike Allen, Facilitator

Desired Project Completion Date: 30 June 1997

Step 2

○ ○ ○ ○ ○

Select the Algorithm Team and Project Leader

```
                    ┌─────────────────┐
                    │  Select algorithm│
      ──────────────▶│ team and project │────────────────▶
                    │     leader       │
                    └─────────────────┘  2
```

In selecting the members of the algorithm team, the steering group must be sure to include not only those who will develop the algorithm, but also those who will assist in the implementation of the completed project. The steering group should choose the team from people who will be using the algorithm on a daily basis. As Deming has repeatedly said, any system improvement must involve the actual system users.[1] These are the individuals who possess actual, or as Deming calls it, "profound" knowledge of the process.

A good team member must have several essential characteristics:

- expertise in the process/treatment activity, as well as daily contact with the treatment activity in question
- an understanding of the value of developing a "best practice" approach
- a willingness to participate actively in developing the algorithm, as well as in marketing the algorithm to skeptical colleagues
- credibility within the profession and among colleagues

(See Resources 2–1 and 2–2 for information on selecting team members.)

The steering group must also designate a project leader for the algorithm effort. In addition to the responsibilities of the other team members, the project leader has several duties that are unique to the position. The primary responsibility of

NOTES

NOTES

the project leader is to guide the algorithm effort and produce a completed algorithm that is consistent with the goals of the organization.

Other specific duties of the project leader include the following:

- acts as liaison between the steering group and the algorithm team. As concerns arise regarding resources and priorities, the project leader works with the steering group to resolve them.
- keeps the algorithm team on task. As many medical practitioners have strong personalities, the ability to keep the team focused and moving forward is of paramount importance.
- keeps the team on schedule.
- resolves conflicts within the team. As conflicts are inevitable, the project leader needs the strength and finesse to deal with them as they occur.
- communicates the progress of the algorithm team within the organization. The project leader acts as the information clearinghouse regarding the progress of the effort.
- assists the facilitator in leading the team meetings.

(See Resource 2–3 on selecting a project leader.)

The second important position designated by the steering group is that of facilitator. Especially in meetings where individuals with strong personalities may have differing opinions of best practice, the position of facilitator is very important. This person should be impartial and should have no stake in the outcome.

The general responsibilities of the facilitator include:

- actively facilitates the algorithm team's adherence to the steps outlined in the five-phase algorithm development flowchart
- works with the project leader to keep the team on task and focused
- ensures that all assignments are clearly understood, documented, acted on, and followed up, if necessary
- manages meetings in a way that achieves decision by consensus
- encourages participation by all members of the team
- chooses the consensus-building techniques that are appropriate for the team

(See Resource 2–4 on selecting a facilitator.)

Other positions that can enhance the algorithm development effort include a recorder (e.g., to keep minutes, do charting) and analyst (e.g., to explain and interpret medical statistical procedures). These individuals need not be full-fledged members of the team; they may function better as temporary team members, participating as the need for their services arises.

NOTE

1. W. E. Deming, *Out of the Crisis* (Cambridge, Massachusetts: Institute of Technology Center for Advanced Engineering Study, 1986).

NOTES

Resource 2–1

○ ○ ○ ○ ○

Selection of Algorithm Team, Project Leader, and Facilitator

Resources 2–2, 2–3, and 2–4 assist the steering group in objectively selecting the individuals who are most likely to succeed as members of the team, as the project leader, and as the facilitator of the algorithm development project.

To use these resources, members of the steering group list all candidates down the left column. Then they rank the candidates from 1 (lowest) to 5 (highest) on each of the criteria selected. Totaling the columns for each candidate provides the steering group with an objective indication of the suitability of each candidate for the position being considered.

The steering group can do this exercise as a group in its meeting, or steering group members can complete it prior to the meeting. Compilation of the results before the meeting allows the steering group to proceed directly into a discussion of the recommendations.

HELPFUL HINTS

- If the steering group decides to rank each candidate during its meeting, it is essential to avoid "groupthink." In group dynamics, the term *groupthink* describes the unwanted influence of one member of the group over another. It can often occur when one member of the group is perceived to be more powerful, or somehow higher, than the other members. A classic example is President John F. Kennedy's decision to invade the Bay of Pigs in Cuba. The President voiced his opinion first. His position of power influenced his advisors, and they proceeded to vote his preference rather than their own. Groupthink can be avoided if the members of the group perform their rankings in private. Once the rankings have been done and written down, they can be shared with the other members of the steering group.

- The project leader and the project facilitator may subsequently recommend the addition, removal, or replacement of a team member, usually because he or she is found not to have the necessary skills to perform the tasks required of the team. The steering group usually supports such a recommendation.

CLINICAL GUIDELINE DEVELOPMENT
Copyright © Aspen Publishers, Inc.

- The steering group has the option of allowing one person to serve as both the project leader and the project facilitator. This step requires caution, however, and the group should monitor the progress of the algorithm team regularly. A person fulfilling both of these positions will have considerable influence over the work and the progress of the algorithm team. The special interest or agenda of a person serving such a dual role can bias the process of developing the algorithm.

Resource 2–2

○ ○ ○ ○

Selection of Algorithm Team Members

Algorithm Title _____ _____ **Date**

Candidates for Algorithm Team	Selection Criteria for Team Members				
	#1	#2	#3	#4	Total
_____					
_____					
_____					
_____					
_____					
_____					
_____					
_____					
_____					
_____					
_____					
_____					
_____					
_____					

Criterion #1 _____ Criterion #3 _____

Criterion #2 _____ Criterion #4 _____

Note: The number of criteria may vary.
Please rank each candidate's qualification for each criterion on a scale of 1 to 5 with 5 being the highest.

Resource 2–3

○ ○ ○ ○ ○

Selection of Algorithm Project Leader

Algorithm Title _____   _____ **Date**

Candidates for Algorithm Project Leader	Selection Criteria for Project Leader						
	#1	#2	#3	#4	#5	#6	Total

Criterion #1 _____   Criterion #4 _____

Criterion #2 _____   Criterion #5 _____

Criterion #3 _____   Criterion #6 _____

Note: The number of criteria may vary.
Please rank each candidate's qualification for each criterion on a scale of
1 to 5 with 5 being the highest.

Resource 2–4

○ ○ ○ ○ ○

Selection of Algorithm Facilitator

Algorithm Title _____   _____ **Date**

Candidates for Algorithm Facilitator	Selection Criteria for Facilitator						
	#1	#2	#3	#4	#5	#6	Total
_____							
_____							
_____							
_____							
_____							
_____							
_____							
_____							
_____							
_____							
_____							

Criterion #1 _____   Criterion #4 _____

Criterion #2 _____   Criterion #5 _____

Criterion #3 _____   Criterion #6 _____

Note: The number of criteria may vary.
Please rank each candidate's qualification for each criterion on a scale of
1 to 5 with 5 being the highest.

Step 3

○ ○ ○ ○ ○

Approve Algorithm
Mission Statement

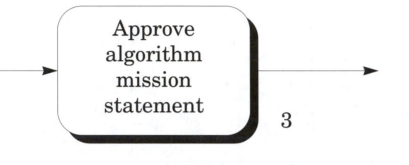

The senior quality council must give its official "stamp of approval" to the algorithm mission statement. In approving the effort, the council ensures that it is consistent with the goals of the organization. The senior quality council also reviews and approves the resources that will be needed both to produce the algorithm and to implement it within the organization.

Before giving the final approval, the senior quality council must be certain that it has given the algorithm team the appropriate message. This is no time for small, minor changes to clinical activities. The team members must understand that the council expects them to discard old paradigms and look at the clinical activity in a new way, to break through organizational barriers, and to establish goals that will stretch the organization's limits and make it stronger. (See Resources 3–1 and 3–2 on council approval of a mission statement.)

Obtaining official approval is the last action involved in the initial stages of the project. The senior quality council and steering group now hand the algorithm development project over to the algorithm team for the beginning of Phase II, Project Definition.

NOTES

Resource 3–1

○ ○ ○ ○ ○

Approval of Algorithm Mission Statement by Senior Quality Council

Resource 3–2 is an organizational checklist to assist the senior quality council in assessing the algorithm's impact upon the organization. The steering group can be assigned this responsibility if its members share the same organizational information as the members of the senior quality council. This checklist serves as a guide for either group in approving, modifying, postponing, or rejecting the first draft of the mission statement.

HELPFUL HINTS

- The senior quality council must provide information, support, and coaching to all personnel in the steering group and the algorithm team. The council must make it clear that this algorithm has the council's full support and will add value to the organization's goals and strategies.
- It is helpful to review the information on Resource 1–3 concerning the difference between a mission statement and a problem statement.

Resource 3–2

○ ○ ○ ○ ○

Approval of Algorithm Mission Statement by Senior Quality Council: Considerations

Algorithm Title _____

Date _____

1. Does the algorithm project conflict or overlap with other current or near-future organizational efforts?_____
2. Does the algorithm project support other strategic initiatives of the organization?_____
3. Can the organization support the possible utilization of personnel time and other resources in light of all other activities and priorities?_____
4. From the organizational perspective, do the possible benefits outweigh the possible costs associated with the algorithm project?_____
5. Does the algorithm project need to be coordinated with other activities or projects within the organization?_____
6. Are there any concerns that the team needs to address?_____
7. Are there ongoing issues that the senior quality council should be aware of as the algorithm effort progresses? (How and when would that occur?)_____
8. Will the results of this effort assist in the marketing of the organization in any way?_____
9. Will the data produced by this algorithm assist the organization in complying with regulatory agencies or assist medical group purchasers of the organization?_____

Phase II

○ ○ ○ ○ ○

Project Definition

The purpose of Phase II, Project Definition, is to ensure that all team members understand what they are being asked to do in the algorithm development project. By the end of this phase, the team members should understand the issue(s) that led to the algorithm and should be able to identify the needs of the customers and users of the completed algorithm.

The first task in this phase is to schedule a meeting of the project leader, the facilitator, and a member of the steering group. Not only does this meeting provide an opportunity for these individuals to get acquainted but also it fulfills several other purposes:

- The roles of the team leader and the facilitator should be clarified.
- The information forwarded from the steering group should be reviewed.
- The various personalities of the team members should be discussed and a plan formulated as to how the team leader and facilitator can best support each member. As a result of this discussion, team members will be participating and contributing at their optimal levels.
- A plan should be developed to notify the team members of their selection to the team. The notification should include dates and locations of meetings, a copy of the mission statement from the steering group, and general information about clinical algorithms and their role in developing best practice. (Eddy,[1] Margolis,[2] and Gottlieb[3] have provided excellent sources of information.)

The first team meeting should be scheduled far enough in advance to accommodate the schedules of all participants. Team members should receive notification at least 4 to 8 weeks prior to the first meeting. They should be given clear instructions regarding their response to this notification. For example, they should be asked to report conflicts in dates and times of meetings immediately. The project leader and the facilitator can accomplish all these tasks before the team meets for the first time. These two people play indispensable roles in the successful beginning of the algorithm effort.

NOTES

1. D. M. Eddy, Clinical Decision Making: From Theory to Practice. The Challenge, *JAMA* 263(1990): 287–290.
2. C. Z. Margolis, Uses of Clinical Algorithms, *JAMA* 249 (1983): 627–632.
3. L. K. Gottlieb, et al., Clinical Practice Guidelines at an HMO: Development and Implementation in a Quality Improvement Model. *Quality Review Bulletin* 16 (1990): 80–86.

Step 4

○ ○ ○ ○ ○

Hold Start-Up Team Meeting

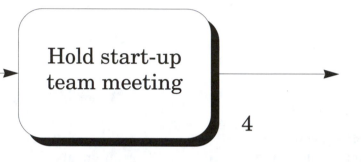

Hold start-up
team meeting

4

When the team meets for the first time, the members learn about the history and background of the issues that led to the algorithm development effort. It is helpful to have a member of the steering group attend the meeting to give an overview of these issues. This person describes the way that the algorithm effort fits with the overall goals of the organization and offers the assistance and support of the steering group in its development. By the conclusion of this discussion, every member should understand the key issues involved in the clinical process being evaluated and the algorithm being developed.

The facilitator then leads the team in a discussion of the algorithm process. The benefits and challenges of developing clinical algorithms (and of standardizing clinical processes) are thoroughly examined. In addition, the information that was sent out to the team members in their selection packets is reviewed.

Although it is unlikely that every team member will be totally convinced of the value of clinical algorithms, this start-up meeting is an opportunity for the project leader and facilitator to introduce the concept and discuss the importance of algorithms in the clinical practice of the organization. Obviously, the more "buy-in" each member has, the more successful the algorithm development effort will be. A certain amount of skepticism in the initial phases of the effort is to be expected, however, and may even help to keep the early discussion balanced.

NOTES

The facilitator also talks the team through the 23 steps of the algorithm development flowchart. This explanation need not be an in-depth discussion of any of the steps, but it gives the team members an idea of the task ahead of them. It also gives the members some assurance that the algorithm development project is a step-by-step process that will produce tangible results.

Finally, the team should make arrangements for the next five or six meeting dates. It is important to clarify and discuss times of meetings, locations, and scheduling conflicts at the first meeting so that they do not become continual sources of frustration for everyone involved. (See Resources 4–1 through 4–4 for assistance with the start-up meeting.)

NOTES

Resource 4–1

○ ○ ○ ○ ○

Start-Up Team Meeting

By being fully prepared and organized at the first meeting of the algorithm team, the facilitator instills confidence in the team members and gets the project off on the right foot. It is the responsibility of the facilitator to develop an agenda for the start-up meeting of the algorithm team that is consistent with the algorithm flowchart. Resource 4–2 is a sample agenda. The general format used in this sample agenda can be beneficial throughout the process. It helps to provide structure and to convince the members that there is a logical "road map" to the final destination.

The use of a checklist to organize a meeting is beneficial to even the most experienced leader or facilitator. Review of a checklist such as that shown in Resource 4–3 prior to the start-up meeting allows the algorithm team to proceed with the fewest possible distractions.

HELPFUL HINTS

- In the opening comments, the facilitator sets the tone for each meeting. The project is updated, and the members are apprised of the project's current status. This is also a time to give any pertinent updates or make assignments that will be discussed later in the meeting. The meeting must not be allowed to get off track during this time of brief remarks, however.

- A member of the steering group or senior quality council should give an overview of the algorithm project. This usually includes the history and background of the algorithm, the way the algorithm fits with the overall goals of the organization, the expectations, and the constraints placed on the algorithm team. Team members should have an opportunity to ask questions and discuss any concerns.

- To help team members learn more about each other, the facilitator asks each member:
  1. name
  2. specialty
  3. years associated with the organization
  4. specific expectations for the algorithm team[*]

5. any questions or concerns about the project[*]
6. potential causes of failure of this project[*]
7. something most people do not know about him or her.

- The assignment sheet (Resource 4–1) is explained. Its purpose is to clarify all commitments made during the meeting.

- Groundrules, the norms expected of each member of the team, make it possible to conduct each meeting in an efficient manner, which, in turn, optimizes the team's chances of success. Sample groundrules for algorithm teams include the following:

  1. A team member who is going to be late to a meeting must call the leader or facilitator by a specific time.
  2. Team members are willing to be influenced.
  3. Side conversations are not allowed.
  4. Conflicts and disagreements are O.K.
  5. Meetings will be canceled if less than 80% of the team can attend.

- After a brief review of the structured approach to algorithm development, it is beneficial to discuss the reasons for standardizing clinical processes. The leader and facilitator can refer to any of several articles in medical journals that will help in this discussion.

- Charting the key insights gained from any information provided to the team is helpful. These insights can come from any source, such as the steering group or the algorithm selection process. Caution is essential, however, to ensure that the team does not attempt to get too far ahead of itself in this time of discussion. The purpose of this exercise is to reinforce the learning already made by the team.

- Because clinicians often have difficulty scheduling time away from patients, it is not usually easy to schedule meetings. It is best to forecast the total number of meetings and to schedule them all at this time. If it becomes apparent that all of the scheduled meetings are not necessary, they can be easily canceled.

---

[*]It would be helpful to have someone record these responses on a chartboard.

Resource 4–2

○ ○ ○ ○ ○

Start-Up Meeting: Sample Agenda

_____   _____
Algorithm Title   **Date**

Name of Organization _____

Title of Algorithm Project _____

Agenda–date _____

I. Opening Comments (Project Leader/Project Facilitator)
  A. Review today's agenda and overview of roles. (Facilitator)
  B. Give "charge" to team. (Steering Group or Senior Quality Council Member.)
     1. Review history and background of issues leading to the initiation of this algorithm development effort.
     2. Discuss how the algorithm fits with the overall goals of the organization.
     3. Clarify steering group/organizational expectations and constraints for this effort. Address initial questions and concerns of team for the steering group/quality council.
  C. Introduce team members and identify expectations. (Facilitator)
  D. Determine meeting dates, time, and location of all meetings.

II. Overview of the Algorithm Development Process (Facilitator)
  A. Discuss benefits and challenges of developing algorithms.
  B. Explain assignment sheet and develop groundrules.
  C. Review the 23-step algorithm development flowchart.

III. Review Initial Data and Information Regarding Algorithm Selection Process (Project Leader/Project Facilitator)

IV. Determination of Actions (Facilitator)
  A. Review assignments and agenda for next meeting.
  B. Determine location/time for next five or six meetings.

Resource 4–3

○ ○ ○ ○ ○

Start-Up Meeting: Checklist

_____   _____

Algorithm Title   **Date**

___ Meeting room free from distractors.

___ Table so all members can comfortably sit and see each other.

___ Enough chairs for all members and steering group guests. (Remove extra chairs to avoid unnecessary splitting of group.)

___ Knowledge of location of rest rooms and telephone.

___ Packets (project binders) for each member, including initial data and information relating to algorithm effort, background medical journal articles on standardization of clinical practice and the rationale of development of algorithms, copy of the 23-step algorithm flowchart and assignment sheet, and list of names and ways to contact other team members.

___ Flip chart easel and chart paper.

___ Felt-tipped pens and tape to hang chart paper on walls.

___ Overhead projector, if needed, for initial presentations.

___ Coffee and refreshments.

___ Meal, if necessary.

___ Start-up meeting agenda precharted and hung on easel.

___ Knowledge of heating and cooling mechanisms for room.

___ Plan to handle telephone messages.

Resource 4–4

○ ○ ○ ○ ○

Start-Up Meeting: Assignment Sheet

Algorithm Title _____ **Date** _____

Attendees _____ _____

_____ _____

_____ _____

Who	*When*	*What*

Step 5

○ ○ ○ ○ ○

Brainstorm Symptoms and Draft/Revise Problem Statement

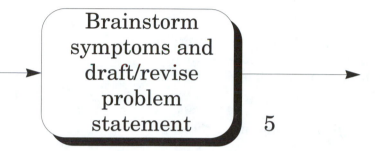

All members of the algorithm development team must understand the clinical process in question from the perspective of every other member. Often, personnel in one department are acutely aware of their problems with a treatment activity, but have no understanding of the inefficiencies or difficulties experienced by personnel in other departments who must deal with the same patient or diagnosis. By the end of the brainstorming session held in step 5, every member of the team should have a more global perspective from which to view the issues that led to the algorithm effort. This new perspective will help the team members write/revise the problem statement.

Before the actual brainstorming session begins, the facilitator should ensure that all team members understand the differences between symptoms and causes. (If a team member does not have a medical background, the facilitator may have to spend some time on this distinction.) To get at the symptoms of a problem-laden clinical process, the facilitator asks such questions as, what is happening to you or to the patient that is outward evidence that this clinical process is not efficient?

During the brainstorming session, the facilitator encourages every team member to make observations and express opinions about the process. The goal is for everyone to hear and understand all perspectives. (See Resources 5–1 and 5–2 for information on brainstorming symptoms.)

NOTES

When all symptoms have been listed, general themes should be identified. It may be necessary to clarify some of the comments and to combine similar symptoms into more general issues. From these general themes, the team can draft/revise the problem statement.

In general, the problem statement should have certain characteristics. It should

- simply state the problem
- contain no suggested or implied solutions
- avoid placing blame
- deal with issues that can be measured, or quantified, rather than opinions.

The problem statement is usually written in a way that describes what is occurring and how it affects patients and/or staff in a quantifiable way. The general format for a problem statement and an example are as follows:

Currently,...(*this is happening*), resulting in...(*these quantifiable symptoms*).

Currently, our treatment of patients diagnosed with shoulder dysfunction varies widely, resulting in decreased reimbursement levels, longer periods of time for patient treatment, variation in scheduling follow-up appointments with support staff, delays in patients returning to work, and decreased patient satisfaction.

NOTES

Resource 5–1

○ ○ ○ ○ ○

Brainstorming Symptoms and Drafting a Problem Statement

Planning ahead can make the difference between success and failure in a brainstorming session. The challenge is to provide an atmosphere for an open, freewheeling, "anything goes" session, while still directing the group's energy toward a meaningful end product. Following these guidelines helps to ensure that the identified problem statement will meet the criteria discussed earlier in the text.

The best setting for a brainstorming session is a group meeting. The facilitator should identify in advance any materials that the group will need in the session and bring them to the meeting—along with enthusiasm and patience. If a group meeting is not feasible, the Delphi method may be helpful. In this method, a questionnaire is sent to each team member. The project leader obtains the answers, has the information collated, and distributes it to team members for the next meeting in formulating a problem statement.

HELPFUL HINT

- The methods utilized to gain input from each team member are limited only by the imagination of the facilitator. These methods can include a simple "going around the table" for input, or can be a creative game such as the following:

  Each team member starts with 10 tokens. Each time a person offers an idea, he or she can give one token to another person of his or her choice. The member with the fewest tokens at the end of the brainstorming session receives a reward.

Resource 5–2

○ ○ ○ ○ ○

Brainstorming Symptoms and Drafting a Problem Statement: Questionnaire

_____   _____

Algorithm Title   **Date**

1. What is happening to you or the patient that is outward evidence that this clinical process/treatment activity is not efficient? _____

   _____

   _____

2. How does the patient view this clinical procedure/treatment activity? _____

   _____

   _____

3. What are the symptoms (not causes)? _____

   _____

   _____

4. What symptoms best exemplify that the clinical process is less than optimal? _____

   _____

   _____

5. Please state the problem in the following format: Currently,...(*this is happening*), resulting in...(*these quantifiable symptoms*). _____

   _____

   _____

Step 6

○ ○ ○ ○ ○

Assess Patient Needs

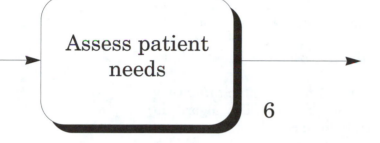

Assess patient needs

6

Once the clinicians have identified the problem(s) involved with the particular clinical process in question, they must assess the needs of the patients involved. The clinicians must think how patients are treated and affected as they proceed through the clinical process.

An assessment of patient needs is necessary to ensure that the outcomes produced by the algorithm being developed will meet the needs of the patients. Throughout the remainder of the algorithm development process, the team must continually refer back to the patient needs. As the team successfully completes each step, it must keep these needs in mind.

Certain needs of all patients are considered fundamental: competency on the part of the clinician, timeliness of care, courtesy on the part of the clinician and staff, and respect as a unique individual. In the past, it was assumed that competency of the clinician is the most important need of the patient. Recently, however, another fundamental patient need has been recognized; this need is so strong that it supersedes all others. The patient needs to have a *trusting relationship* (or partnership) with the clinician. For years, patients have not experienced such a relationship.

The typical relationship between a clinician and a patient has resembled that of a parent and a child. The clinician has told the patient what the problem is and what the clinician is going to do to make the patient better. In the last decade of the twentieth century, this model is long outdated. Patients

NOTES

are much more educated concerning their conditions and much more eager to participate in the decisions about their treatment. In addition, third-party payers are making decisions that affect the patient's financial well-being. With the combined pressures of having an illness and paying for its treatment, patients' need to have a trusting relationship with the clinician is of even greater importance. Patients must feel that the clinician has their best interest at heart, and the clinician must communicate that to the patient at every opportunity.

To assess patient needs for algorithm development, the facilitator first asks the team to identify the patient population that this treatment activity affects. The team members are then asked, "What do you perceive to be the fundamental needs of these patients?" After a discussion of the needs suggested, the team has to ask itself, "Do we feel confident that this is an accurate representation of the patients' needs?" If the answer is yes, the team should discuss, examine, and prioritize the needs that have been listed.

A note of caution is warranted here. Clinicians often *think* they instinctively know the needs of their patients. The algorithm team may be well served, however, to form a task force to survey the patients themselves to determine their needs. Many health care organizations are already conducting surveys to determine patient satisfaction. A member of the team should contact the patient relations department for information that may be of value. Any current patient survey may need only slight modifications to meet the requirements of the algorithm team.

Finally, the team may have to examine the clinical process to determine if it involves more than one distinct patient population. For example, to address the orthopaedic and rehabilitation needs of patients with hip fractures that required open reduction/internal fixation, it is necessary to differentiate between patients who were ambulatory before surgery and those who were not. Similarly, the physical therapy needs of a 17-year-old athlete who has sustained a complete tear of the anterior cruciate ligament in the knee may differ from those of a 60-year-old person with a sedentary life style.

If such differences exist, the team must decide which patient population the algorithm will address. If it becomes necessary to narrow the scope of the algorithm in this fashion, the team must notify the steering group for approval. (See Resources 6–1 and 6–2 for assessing patient needs.)

Resource 6–1

○ ○ ○ ○ ○

Patient Needs Assessment

Having developed a problem statement, the algorithm team should complete a patient needs assessment. The purpose of this step is to ensure that the algorithm will produce outcomes that meet the specific needs of patients. Quality is ultimately defined by the "customers."

HELPFUL HINTS

- Although the patient needs assessment is best done as a group activity, time or scheduling may necessitate use of the Delphi method.
- If the confidence level discussed in Step 4 is not high, a task force can gain additional information from patients by survey, interview, or other means. If the organization has a patient relations department, the team may be able to make use of that resource.

Resource 6–2

○ ○ ○ ○ ○

Patient Needs Assessment: Considerations

_____   _____
Algorithm Title   **Date**

1. Which patient population is affected by this treatment activity? _____

   _____

   _____

2. What are the fundamental needs of these patients? Please prioritize. _____

   _____

   _____

3. How confident are you that this is an accurate representation of the patient needs? _____

   _____

   _____

4. Is there more than one distinct patient population involved? If so, which population will be specifically addressed by this algorithm? _____

   _____

   _____

Step 7

○ ○ ○ ○ ○

Define Expected Outcomes

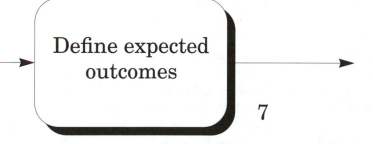

Define expected
outcomes

7

The algorithm team received proposed expected outcomes in the initial draft of the mission statement from the steering group. After its careful assessment of patient needs, however, the team may want to revise or change the expected outcomes.

The successful completion of Step 7 is not as easy as it may first appear. There are three categories in which expected outcomes may be included:

1. *Patient satisfaction measures.* This is probably the most obvious category, as the algorithm team has just thoroughly assessed the needs of the patients involved. Measures in this category will simply focus on such questions as, Has patient satisfaction improved after the algorithm has been implemented?

2. *Clinical process outcome/performance measures.* This category will deal with such questions as, Has the quality of care of the patient improved because of the algorithm? Have patients recovered in less time? Have more patients been accurately diagnosed in a shorter period of time? Clinical process performance measures deal with optimal care and the patient outcomes resulting from that optimal care. Examples of these measures include rate of re-admission, perceived level of pain following treatment, distance walked without assistance, and length of hospital stay.

NOTES

3. *Clinical compliance and efficiency (in-process) measures.* This final category will involve measures of the level of accuracy demonstrated by the clinicians who use the algorithm. Is the algorithm being strictly followed? If so, has the algorithm increased the efficiency with which patients are now being treated? If the algorithm is not being followed, where is it breaking down? Examples of these measures are the number of times a certain diagnostic test was ordered, the number of times outside consultation was requested, or the number of follow-up telephone calls made. All such measures will be stated in ratios, compared to the total number of patients.

Choosing from these three categories, the team defines the expected outcomes of the finished algorithm. Once the outcomes have been defined, the team must propose ways to determine if the outcomes are being achieved. This task is of the utmost importance in measuring the ultimate effectiveness of an algorithm.

During Step 7, the measures are proposed and briefly discussed. The outcomes and clinical indicators used to measure results are thoroughly discussed and quantified during Steps 11 and 12 and Steps 20 and 21. (See Resources 7–1 through 7–2 for assistance in defining expected outcomes. Resource 7–3 illustrates the algorithm measurement system.)

NOTES

Resource 7–1

○ ○ ○ ○ ○

Definition of Expected Outcomes

Presenting an overview of the algorithm measurement system helps the team understand the importance of Step 7 and the use of the team's output in later steps.

HELPFUL HINTS

- After completing the algorithm measurement system, the team should review each expected outcome proposed by the steering group.
- Although the expected outcomes should be clear to all team members, it is not necessary to develop the final clinical indicators and measures at this time.
- It is desirable to have at least one expected outcome in each of the three categories. The team should seriously consider adding or modifying expected outcomes so that all three categories are represented.
- All expected outcomes should ultimately meet the identified needs of the patient, as identified in Resource 6–2.
- The team must report any changes or revisions in the original expected outcomes to the steering group.

Resource 7–2

○ ○ ○ ○ ○

Definition of Expected Outcomes: Questionnaire

_____   _____

Algorithm Title   **Date**

1. List the expected outcomes as found in the mission statement of the steering group.

   _____

   _____

   _____

2. As written, are the outcomes clearly understood?

   _____

   _____

   _____

3. For each outcome, indicate the appropriate category:

   1. Patient satisfaction measures

   2. Clinical process outcome/performance measures

   3. Clinical compliance and efficiency measures

4. For each expected outcome, identify the fundamental need of the patient that the outcome addresses.

   _____

   _____

   _____

   _____

5. Revise any expected outcome, if necessary.

Resource 7–3

○ ○ ○ ○ ○

Algorithm Measurement System

Steering Group
Defines
"Expected Outcomes" (**Step 1**)

↓

Algorithm Team
Refines
"Expected Outcomes" (**Step 7**)

↓

Algorithm Team
Clarifies
"Expected Clinical Outcomes" (**Step 11**)

↓

Algorithm Team
Determines
"Clinical Indicators" (**Step 12**)

↓

Algorithm Team
Finalizes
"Ongoing Measure" (**Step 20**)

↓

Algorithm Team
Develops
"Monitoring Methodology" (**Step 21**)

↓

Phase III

○ ○ ○ ○ ○

Algorithm Development

By Phase III, the algorithm development team has a clear definition of the problem and a clear understanding of the issues that are signaling the need for an algorithm. The team members have built a consensus concerning the specific products (outputs) to be generated by the algorithm process and the results (outcomes) to be expected from the implementation of the actual algorithm. Equally important, the team is aware of the effect that this algorithm will have on the needs of the patient. At this point the team is ready to begin the step-by-step approach of building an algorithm.

Step 8

○ ○ ○ ○ ○

Assess Clinical User Needs

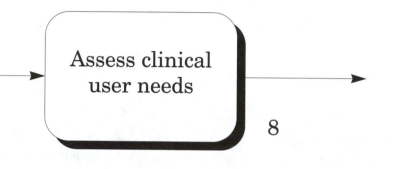

Assess clinical
user needs

8

Absolutely critical for the effective implementation of a clinical algorithm is an assessment of clinical user needs. Unless the needs of the individuals who will actually use the algorithms on a day-to-day basis are assessed and addressed during algorithm development, full compliance is highly unlikely. Everyone who is a potential user of the algorithm must feel that his or her concerns have been heard and addressed so that there is a unanimous "buy-in" on the finished product.

If the algorithm team is representative of all the potential users, it may be adequate to have the individual members of the team list and discuss their concerns regarding the algorithm project. If it is preferable to obtain input from every potential user, the team can develop a simple survey to accomplish this task. (See Resources 8–1 and 8–2 for an algorithm development survey.)

A survey such as the one in Resource 8–2 gives the algorithm team a definite sense of what is important to the users of the clinical algorithm.

As the respondents list their concerns, they provide answers such as:

- "must be easy to use"
- "must be cost-effective"
- "cannot add staff"
- "increase confidence in my decision-making ability"
- "cannot add to paperwork."

NOTES

All specific comments such as these help focus the team and begin the buy-in process for everyone involved. Having the respondents rank their answers further assists the team in the prioritization of issues. (See Resources 8–3 and 8–4 for information on tracking the algorithm development survey.)

Resource 8–1

○ ○ ○ ○ ○

Assessment of Clinical User Needs

The team can make long-term changes in the organization's clinical practice only by identifying the "real world" needs of the people who will be using the algorithm. Contacting all algorithm users regarding their specific needs encourages "buy-in" from everyone.

HELPFUL HINTS

- The team should list all the potential algorithm users within the organization.
- It is helpful to provide a means of easily returning the survey (e.g., a self-addressed stamped envelope).
- The team should make sure that the supervisors of the personnel being surveyed are aware of the algorithm development process.
- The team should keep track of the forms sent out and received.

Resource 8–2

○ ○ ○ ○ ○

Assessment of Clinical User Needs: Survey

_____   _____

Algorithm Title   **Date**

1. A team has been assembled to develop an algorithm regarding the clinical process noted above. The following personnel have been identified as process users:

   _____   _____

   _____   _____

   _____   _____

   _____   _____

   _____   _____

2. It is critical that all potential users of this algorithm are identified. Please list any additional clinicians who may be affected by this algorithm:

   _____   _____

   _____   _____

   _____   _____

3. What does this algorithm have to accomplish to make it usable and effective?

   ___ Enhance sensitivity of screening

   ___ Speed up process

   ___ Require less paperwork

   ___ Involve less "shuffling" of the patient

   ___ Other (Explain)

4. What would it take for you to accept the algorithm?

   ___ It would have to decrease the uncertainty of my decisions.

   ___ I would have to be able to understand the algorithm.

___ It would have to make sense to me.

___ It would allow me to spend more time with my patients.

___ It would cut down on rework, inefficiencies, etc.

___ Other (Explain)

5. Please list your concerns about the algorithm process. Place an X by the two concerns that you feel are the most important.

_____

_____

_____

_____

_____

_____

_____

_____

_____

_____

Thank you for your input. Please return this survey to _____no later than _____.

We appreciate your support and continued assistance with this project.

Resource 8–3

○ ○ ○ ○ ○

Tracking of Algorithm Development Survey

The time spent in identifying and contacting all clinicians affected by the algorithm will be paid back many times over. The more the potential algorithm users feel that their input is important, the better their ultimate "buy-in."

HELPFUL HINTS

- Interviewing department heads and supervisors is a good place to begin the process of identifying potential algorithm users. It is also an opportunity to gain support from these individuals.
- One person should be in charge of tracking the surveys and keeping the master list of all clinicians who have been contacted.
- A personal contact to follow up ensures a prompt response and provides an opportunity to express appreciation for taking the time to fill out the survey.
- There need be no concern about "overthanking" the people who are returning the surveys. The team must have their "buy-in" for the algorithm to be successful.

CLINICAL GUIDELINE DEVELOPMENT
Copyright © Aspen Publishers, Inc.

Resource 8–4

○ ○ ○ ○ ○

Algorithm Development Survey: Tracking Form

Algorithm Title   **Date**

Algorithm User	Date Survey Sent	Date Survey Returned	Person Who Contacted User	Date Contacted

Step 9

○ ○ ○ ○ ○

Review Current Practices and Identify Learnings

```
Review current
practices and
identify learnings
                    9
```

The algorithm development team must evaluate what is currently happening in the clinical process. This is not the time for team members to determine the optimal process, or what should be happening, but, rather, a time for the team to evaluate the existing process.

This step can be a valuable learning experience as various team members describe facets of the process that may be unfamiliar to the others. Team members share what is working well in the process and what is not. They also identify areas of re-work during this step.

Finally, a thorough review of the current process will expose the uncertainties and variations that occur from person to person, from day to day. The completion of this step should convince everyone involved that it is beneficial to standardize the key processes of the clinical practice.

To determine what is currently happening in a process, the team should develop a high-level flowchart. This type of flowchart lists the major events of the process as it is being practiced at the present time. It is a broad view of the process and does not detail every component of each event. There are three major cautions for Step 9:

1. Remember to look at the process as it is happening now.
2. Stick with a flowchart, and do not attempt to develop the algorithm during this step.
3. Recognize that there is likely to be significant variation and uncertainty in the process, if there is a process at all.

NOTES

While constructing the flowchart of current practices, the team should continually ask the following questions:

- What do we agree upon as essential components of the process?
- What are the areas of disagreement?
- Where are there variations in the process among staff?
- Where is there confusion during the process?

By asking questions such as these, the team is able to identify, discuss, and list the learnings gleaned from the flowcharting procedures. (See Resources 9–1 through 9–3 for assistance in reviewing current practices and developing a flowchart.)

NOTES

Resource 9–1

○ ○ ○ ○ ○

Review of Current Practices

High-level flowcharts help to identify areas of re-work, break-downs, and needless variations. The insights concerning the inadequacies and inefficiencies of the current clinical process/treatment activity that come from such a flowchart allow the team to address the areas of concern and make appropriate changes in the algorithm.

HELPFUL HINTS

- Clearly identifying the Start and Stop points of the clinical process will keep the algorithm from growing out of control in either size or scope.
- A high-level flowchart deals with only major events in the clinical process; a detailed, complex algorithm of the current process requires unnecessary expenditures of time and energy by the team.
- During the flowchart process, it is not uncommon for the team to be uncertain about what is actually happening during every step of the clinical activity. Often, those areas of uncertainty are the very reasons that an algorithm has been proposed. On the flowchart, these areas of uncertainty are represented by a cloud symbol.

CLINICAL GUIDELINE DEVELOPMENT
Copyright © Aspen Publishers, Inc.

Resource 9–2

○ ○ ○ ○ ○

Review of Current Practices:
Flowchart Process

---------------------------------   ---------------------------------
Algorithm Title   **Date**

What is the Start point of this algorithm? _____

What is the Stop point? _____

What are the major steps that currently occur during this
clinical process?

Major Step 1. _____

   Decisions made during this step:

   _____

   _____

Major Step 2. _____

   Decisions made during this step:

   _____

   _____

Major Step 3. _____

   Decisions made during this step:

   _____

   _____

Major Step 4. _____

   Decisions made during this step:

   _____

   _____

Major Step 5. _____

    Decisions made during this step:

_____

_____

Major Step 6. _____

    Decisions made during this step:

_____

_____

In the space below, draw the final version of a flowchart of the clinical process as it is currently happening:

List the areas of potential re-work, breakdowns, or needless variations.

_____

_____

_____

List any other key insights from this step.

_____

_____

_____

Resource 9–3

● ● ● ● ●

Review of Current Practices: Sample High-Level Flowchart

Emergency Room Patient with Traumatic Headache

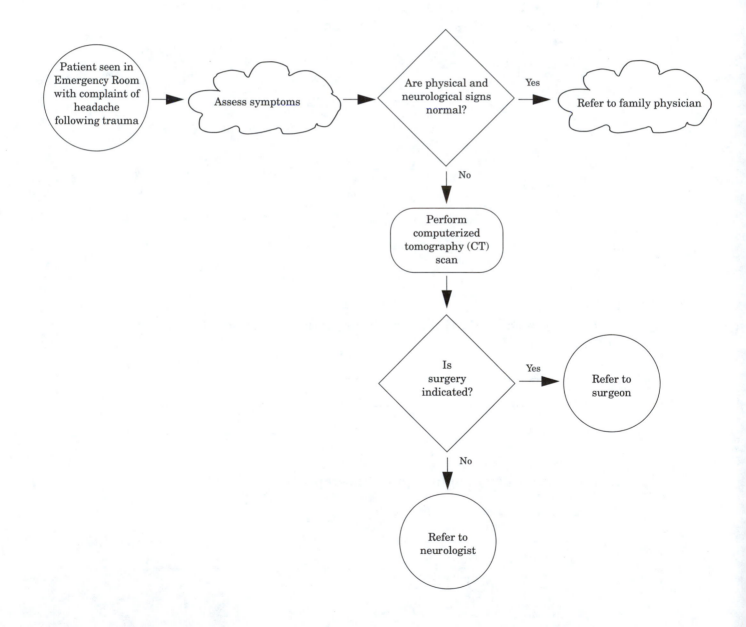

Step 10

○ ○ ○ ○ ○

Review Literature Regarding "Best Practice" Based on Reliable Research

> Review literature regarding "best practice" based on reliable research

10

Once the algorithm development team members have an accurate understanding of what clinicians in their organization are currently doing in the treatment activity, it is time to investigate how others are performing the same activity. The main purpose of this step is education. The team gathers information about new concepts and methods from people who are considered experts in the field. This information will help resolve the areas of disagreements identified in Step 9.

For algorithms relating to clinical practices, the most effective way to conduct a literature review is to use the information service of a hospital or university. By using a key word or phrase, the service can usually provide a list of all the publications about the topic under consideration.

As with any review of literature, the team must be cognizant of the methodology used in the studies reported. Because some journals, for example, publish reports of studies that do not meet rigid research standards and use scientific methods, the reviewer must always consider the research methods used before accepting at face value the conclusions presented in the report. Also, the reviewer should check to see if a corporation has sponsored a publication that is favorable to a specific product. Although this does not automatically make a study useless, the reviewer should be aware of any possible sponsor bias. (See Resources 10–1 and 10–2 for reviewing literature.)

The way that the algorithm team decides to conduct the literature search is up to the individual members of the team. If

NOTES

the clinical process can be easily divided into distinct topics, the team leader may assign all members a different topic. It may be easier, however, to assign one member the task of obtaining the pertinent publications and then to divide them equally among the members for review and discussion.

There may be few, if any, good publications on some aspects of a clinical process. In these instances, the team can try to find out if there is a clinic/hospital/practice anywhere in the world that is performing the process better than anyone else in the medical field. If so, a team member can contact the institution to obtain "benchmark" information.

No matter how the team obtains the information involved in Step 10, it is once again essential to discuss the key learnings from all the information. The team must decide what portions of the information are pertinent to the clinical process being evaluated.

NOTES

Resource 10–1

○ ○ ○ ○ ○

Literature Review

Review of benchmark literature often requires assignments to several of the team members. Various publications can be handed out to members for review and report. Discussion of critical elements of each article will help to determine the "best practice".

HELPFUL HINTS

- Each reference should be evaluated on a separate form and the key learnings identified. Key learnings are best reported as short, "bullet" statements. Highlighted copies of the reviewed literature may also be included for the team discussion.
- The methodology of each study should be evaluated for validity and reliability. Inadequate methodology should be noted. Methodology is often indicated in the abstracts for ease of reviewing and reporting.
- Publications and follow-up references that come to light from them should be listed.

Resource 10–2

○ ○ ○ ○ ○

Literature Review: Considerations

Algorithm Title   **Date**

1. Publication/research being evaluated:

   _____

   _____

2. List the key insights that pertain specifically to the clinical process that is being studied.

   • _____

   • _____

   • _____

   • _____

3. What methodology was used to determine the validity and reliability of the results?

   _____

   _____

4. Are there any sponsors of the research whose products may receive favorable review because of the conclusions of the research? If so, list the products:

   _____

   _____

5. List any references that should be investigated for further information or review.

   _____

   _____

   _____

Step 11

○ ○ ○ ○ ○

Define Clinical Outcomes To Be Achieved

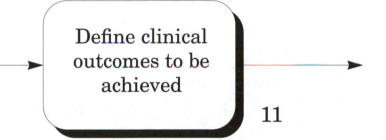

Define clinical outcomes to be achieved

11

A careful examination of the process being evaluated makes it possible to define the patient outcomes expected to result from the clinical algorithm. In Step 7, clinical outcome performance measures were discussed as one of the three categories for expected outcomes of an algorithm. In Step 11, these performance measures are reviewed and examined in more detail. These expected outcome statements must be written in quantifiable, measurable terms that everyone can understand. In developing expected outcomes, the team must ask, "What must happen to the patient for the algorithm to be considered effective?" and "How can we measure the effects on the patient?"

It is difficult to write expected outcome statements that meet the criteria just discussed. If the expected clinical outcome statements are poorly written, however, it is impossible to determine if the algorithm has had a positive impact on the clinical practice in question. Examples of poorly worded statements are "no evidence of respiratory distress," "viable skin graft," or "stable surgical wound."

None of these expected clinical outcome statements indicate whether the algorithm has had the desired effect on patient care. They are subjective and contain no information that can be measured and duplicated — either over time or among clinicians.

Examples of well written expected outcome statements include the following:

NOTES

- "Newborn weight of 2,000 grams or more"
- "Passive knee flexion greater than 90 degrees"
- "Diastolic blood pressure variation less than 30 mm Hg without intravenous hematensive drugs"
- "Total blood cholesterol of 200 mg or less"

All of these examples include information that can be accurately assessed to determine the efficacy of the algorithm. After developing a list of possible expected outcome statements, the team must prioritize them. Completing this evaluation process gives the team members a clearer sense of what needs to be included in the algorithm and what does not. (See Resources 11–1 and 11–2 on defining clinical outcomes.)

The algorithm development team must remember the "charge" of the senior quality council and develop expected clinical outcomes that stretch the limits of the organization. Often clinicians view a clinical activity in a certain manner because that's the way it has always been done. Developing an algorithm requires the team members to throw out such paradigms and begin the process with no preconceived notions. Changes in the way health care is delivered and reimbursed demand major revisions in the way organizations develop their vision of "best practice."

NOTES

Resource 11–1

○ ○ ○ ○ ○

Definition of Clinical Outcomes

Like "quality of care," "best practice" is ultimately defined by the customer or patient. Thus, the algorithm development team must view the results of the clinical process/treatment activity through the eyes of the patient. Changing the clinical practice in a way that does not positively affect patient outcome is a waste of time and resources, especially in this demanding environment of health care reform. The use of a form such as that shown in Resource 11–2 will help the team keep focused on the needs of the patient while choosing the final outcome measures for the algorithm.

HELPFUL HINTS

- Based on the data gathered in the completion of Steps 8, 9, and 10 of the algorithm flowchart, the team may have to modify the expected outcomes. The team must be positive that the effects on the patient can be measured.

- The value of each clinical outcome can be prioritized in relation to the other clinical outcomes stated. The team performs this step after completing questions 1 through 4 on Resource 11–2.

- The team must keep the following question in mind: What must happen to the patient for the algorithm to be considered successful? It is all too easy for clinicians to focus on the needs of clinicians instead of those of the patient.

- After completing a form for all expected outcomes, the team members must choose which measures to keep so that the team can advance to the next step—identifying clinical indicators.

Resource 11–2

○ ○ ○ ○ ○

Definition of Clinical Outcomes: Prioritization

_____   _____
Algorithm Title   **Date**

1. List the expected outcomes already identified. _____
   _____
   _____

2. Describe what happens to the patient when the expected clinical outcome has been achieved. _____
   _____
   _____

3. Modify any expected outcome statements that need "fine tuning." _____
   _____
   _____

4. List the units of measure for each expected outcome. _____
   _____
   _____

5. Prioritize the expected outcomes in relation to their importance to the patient. _____
   _____
   _____

Step 12

○ ○ ○ ○ ○

Define Possible Clinical Indicators

The development of well written statements of quantifiable expected outcomes is a prerequisite for the development of indicators that monitor whether the expected outcomes are being achieved. In completing Step 12, the team members establish criteria that indicate the effectiveness of the algorithm on the patient.

Again, the indicators must be described in quantifiable terms so that clinicians can generate data to determine the patient's improvement (thus measuring the effectiveness of the algorithm).

The Joint Commission on Accreditation of Healthcare Organizations has included a discussion of other attributes of clinical indicators.[1]

- Validity: the extent to which the indicator accomplishes its purpose. Does the indicator identify the process, or situation, being examined?

- Face validity: the extent to which the indicator makes sense. Can the informed user understand the indicator?

- Sensitivity: the extent to which the indicator is able to identify all aspects of a particular process. Are there areas of the process that the indicator does not monitor?

- Specificity: the extent to which the indicator is able to identify only those areas of a process in which problems exist. Does the indicator measure more than what the team wants it to measure?

NOTES

An indicator expresses information as a ratio of events within a defined universe. When the ratio is arranged as a fraction, the numerator is the number of times (or patients) the indicator event occurs; the denominator is the total number of patients who have the condition or procedure that the indicator is assessing.

The clinical indicator must be specific as to the type of patient, condition, or diagnosis. It is important to avoid such words as stable or controlled because taken alone, these words do not have measurable, quantifiable meanings.

Following are examples of indicators that meet these criteria:

$$\frac{\text{Number of patients voiding at least 800 cc of urine within first 24 hours following laminectomy}}{\text{Number of patients undergoing laminectomy}}$$

$$\frac{\text{Number of total hip replacement patients not independently ambulating with a walker more than 100 feet at time of discharge}}{\text{Number of patients undergoing total hip replacement}}$$

$$\frac{\text{Number of hysterectomy patients requiring readmission within 72 hours after discharge}}{\text{Number of hysterectomy patients discharged}}$$

These examples are valid, sensitive, specific, and quantifiable. The use of any of these indicators would help to determine if the relevant algorithm is effective and is achieving the expected outcomes that the team has established. (See Resources 12–1 and 12–2 for information on evaluating clinical indicators.)

NOTE

1. Joint Commission on Accreditation of Healthcare Organizations, Characteristics of Clinical Indicators, *Quality Review Bulletin* 15(1989):330–339.

Resource 12–1

○ ○ ○ ○ ○

Clinical Indicators Evaluation

Indicators that monitor whether expected outcomes have been achieved are crucial to the evaluation and improvement of a clinical process. If well written, quantifiable expected clinical outcome statements were developed with Resource 11–2, then the development of meaningful indicators is the next logical step. Resource 12–2 helps to ensure that the team includes all attributes of well written clinical indicators. A new form should be used for each possible clinical indicator.

HELPFUL HINTS

- The team should not attempt to rush through this step. It is surprising how often an organization attempts to measure the effectiveness of an algorithm with poorly written and, therefore, inadequate clinical indicators.
- The whole team should participate in the evaluation of each clinical indicator. Copying the outline of each Resource 12–2 on a large chart board may facilitate a forum of open, critical discussion of the suitability of each indicator.
- If the team is confused or not progressing, the leader may review Step 11.
- After the team has agreed on which clinical indicators may be used, consultation with an "outside expert" may be helpful. This is especially true if any uncertainty remains among team members.
- There is no such thing as a perfect measure. It is not necessary for a measure to meet all criteria; the goal is to develop the best possible indicator.

Resource 12–2

○ ○ ○ ○ ○

Clinical Indicators
Evaluation Sheet

Algorithm Title   **Date**

1. List a clinical outcome. _____
   _____

2. Identify a unit of measure that will determine if the outcome has been achieved. _____

3. Using a ratio of units of measure, identify an indicator that is appropriate for this expected outcome. _____
   _____

4. Does the indicator easily identify the process being examined? (*Validity*) _____
   _____

   What process does it identify?_____
   _____

5. Can all informed users understand the indicator? (*Face Validity*) _____
   _____

6. List the aspect of the clinical process that this indicator identifies. (*Sensitivity*) _____
   _____

7. Does the indicator identify only those areas of the process for which it is intended? (*Specificity*)_____
   _____

   What aspect of the clinical process does this indicator measure?_____
   _____

   What are other aspects of this process that need to be measured by another clinical indicator? _____
   _____

Step 13

○ ○ ○ ○ ○

Identify/Discuss Seed Algorithm

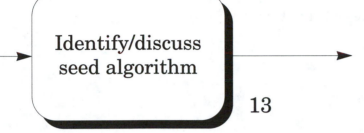

Identify/discuss
seed algorithm

13

"Let's don't re-invent the wheel." It is almost a certainty that someone will express this sentiment either directly or indirectly during the development of a seed algorithm, or starting point, that will eventually become the final product.

As the team reviews the results of the literature search, it will become apparent that other hospitals and clinics are performing the process in a different—perhaps better—manner. It is the responsibility of the algorithm development team to include in the seed algorithm the ideas from the research that, taken together, represent the "best practice" for the users of the algorithm.

Using the benchmark information obtained from the experts in the field and the research accumulated in Step 10, the team extracts the best ideas to be incorporated into the clinical practice of the team and the algorithm users. The key to this process is to adapt the benchmark ideas to the unique situation of the algorithm team and users. The ideas cannot simply be copied directly from one hospital/clinic to another or from one medical practice to another. Every situation is unique with differences in staff, patient population, etc. The algorithm developmental team must recognize that "best practice" refers to the unique characteristics of each medical organization.

The "seed" algorithm is a rough draft of the algorithm process that incorporates the learnings obtained from all of the steps to this point. It is not imperative for the format of the

NOTES

algorithm to be completely accurate or for the symbols to be absolutely correct at each step along the way. It is important, however, for the team to reach consensus as to the overall direction of the algorithm. Upon completion of the seed, the team and the algorithm users will have a document that will allow them to discuss intelligently all the potential steps of the clinical process being evaluated. (See Resources 13–1 and 13–2 for assistance in developing a seed algorithm.)

Because of the difficulty of reaching consensus, it is often helpful for the team to assign one or two members the task of gathering all of the information discussed up to this point and forming a rough draft of the document. As mentioned, the rough draft need not be exact, but it is helpful to follow the standard algorithm format that uses the symbols discussed in Step 14. An example of a seed algorithm is presented in Resource 13–3.

NOTES

Resource 13–1

○ ○ ○ ○ ○

Development of a Seed Algorithm

The development of a seed algorithm by one to two members of the algorithm team can expedite the development of the final algorithm. Resource 13–2 can help in planning an algorithm so that it addresses all major components of the clinical process. The team should remember to use the information obtained from its review of any pertinent literature and contacts (benchmarking).

The seed algorithm should outline enough of the process to facilitate timely completion of the final draft without being so extensive as to limit discussion. The author of the "seed" should be willing to allow for deviation after a thorough discussion of the process by the team.

HELPFUL HINT

- A seed algorithm is only a rough draft and serves as a starting point for discussion. The one or two authors should not get bogged down in details, nor should they be overly protective of this first draft. After a thorough discussion by the full team, there are likely to be many changes or revisions.

Resource 13–2

○ ○ ○ ○ ○

Development of a Seed Algorithm: Planning Form

_____   _____
Algorithm Title   **Date**

What are the key learnings obtained from the literature that pertain to this algorithm? _____

_____

_____

_____

What is the Start point of this algorithm? _____

What is the Stop point? _____

What are the major steps that will occur for this clinical process when the algorithm is performing effectively? Avoid excessive detail.

Major Step 1. _____

   Decisions and component steps made:

   _____

   _____

   _____

   _____

Major Step 2. _____

   Decisions and component steps made:

   _____

   _____

   _____

   _____

Major Step 3. _____

    Decisions and component steps made:

    _____

    _____

    _____

Major Step 4. _____

    Decisions and component steps made:

    _____

    _____

    _____

Major Step 5. _____

    Decisions and component steps made:

    _____

    _____

    _____

Major Step 6. _____

    Decisions and component steps made:

    _____

    _____

    _____

Major Step 7. _____

    Decisions and component steps made:

    _____

    _____

    _____

Major Step 8. _____

    Decisions and component steps made:

    _____

    _____

    _____

Resource 13–3

○ ○ ○ ○ ○

Seed Algorithm

Routine Papanicolaou Screening of Women without History of Cervical Cancer

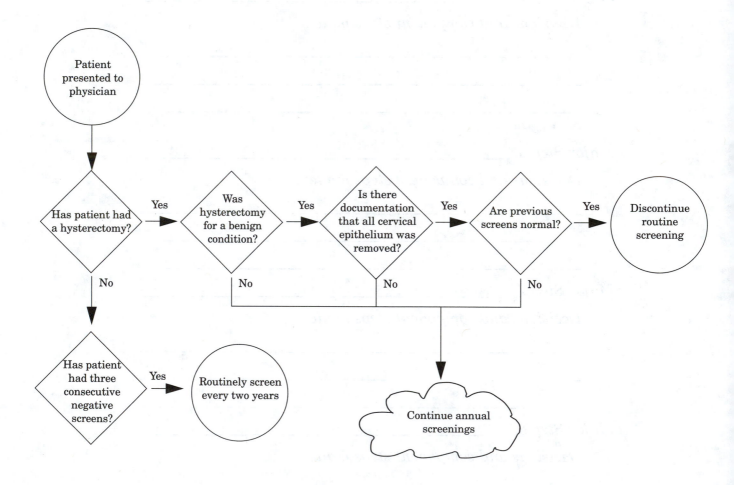

Step 14

○ ○ ○ ○ ○

Develop Algorithm Using Standardized Format

```
              ┌──────────────┐
              │   Develop    │
 ─────────────▶│ algorithm using│──────────────▶
              │ standardized │
              │   format     │
              └──────────────┘  14
```

Throughout the discussions of the first 13 steps, the importance of gaining consensus has been mentioned repeatedly. Nowhere in this entire process is it more important to gain consensus than in Step 14. Consensus does not mean that everyone agrees completely with every aspect of the algorithm. It means that the algorithm users can agree enough with any controversial aspect to be willing to incorporate it into their clinical practice.

Gaining this consensus in a group of medical practitioners can be a difficult and exhausting procedure. The preferable way to achieve consensus is to have all the algorithm users in a room together and have a skilled facilitator lead the group through the entire process.

Another way to gain consensus is by mail. In this approach, the users are sent a copy of the algorithm and instructed to return it by a certain date with their questions and comments. This method is more time efficient in that it does not require a meeting of all clinicians at the same time. There is also much less chance of conflict. The process of sending out, revising, sending out again, revising again, etc., markedly increases the time involved to complete the project, however.

Whatever method they use to gain consensus, the team members now review and refine the seed algorithm into the final product. The first step in constructing the actual algorithm is to agree on the Start/Stop points. When does the process start, and when does it end? Even these seemingly easy decisions occasionally cause animated discussions.

In order for everyone to understand an algorithm, it must be constructed using the format that has been standardized

NOTES

for all algorithms—regardless of the subject matter. Certain symbols signify certain types of activity in all algorithms. The most common are as follows:

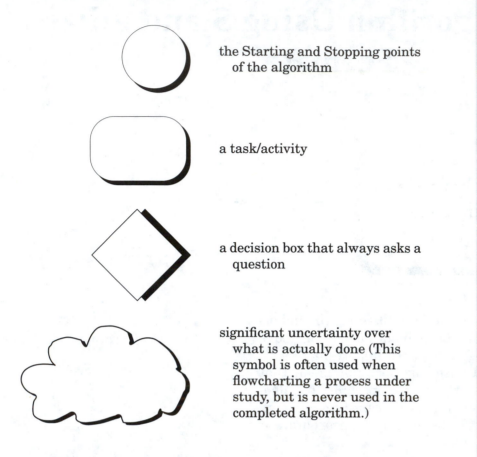

the Starting and Stopping points of the algorithm

a task/activity

a decision box that always asks a question

significant uncertainty over what is actually done (This symbol is often used when flowcharting a process under study, but is never used in the completed algorithm.)

In addition, an algorithm usually flows in a certain direction—either left to right or up and down. The direction depends on the number of boxes used and the type of decisions that must be made throughout the algorithm. After a decision box, the answer yes usually continues along with the flow of the algorithm.

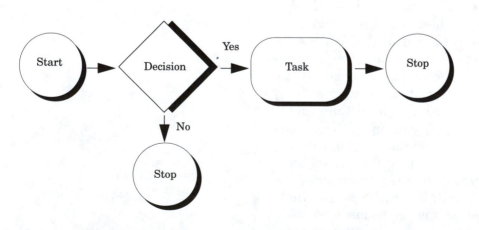

No matter the shape of the symbol, each is numbered at the lower right-hand corner. This notation facilitates discussion of

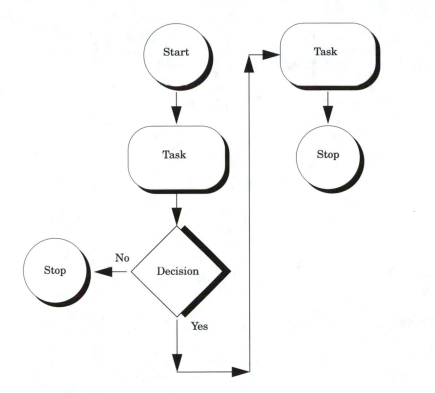

the algorithm by its users who might have a "question about Box 10," for example.

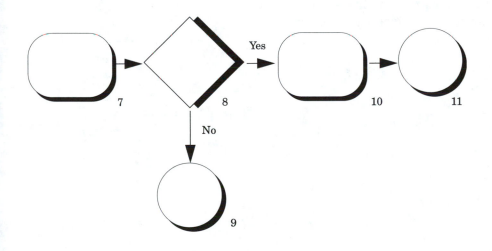

Sometimes, a symbol represents a component of the algorithm that requires further discussion or clarification that cannot be squeezed into a small space. Capital letters placed at the upper right-hand corner of the appropriate symbol can refer the algorithm user to a separate sheet that contains the annotations and the information needed to clarify the information found in the symbol.

Through practice, patience, and the use of this standardized format, the team can develop an algorithm that defines its "best practice." As the algorithm is being finished, the team must

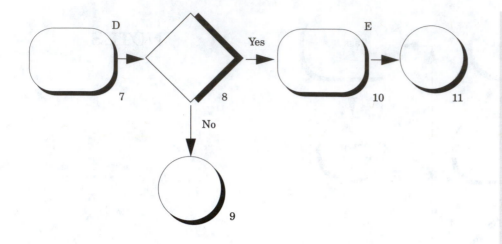

return to the learnings obtained in Steps 6 and 8 for a final check. The members must ask themselves,

- Does this algorithm meet the needs of the patients and of the algorithm users?
- Are there concerns of either group that have not been addressed?
- What must be added to or subtracted from the algorithm for all the needs to be met or exceeded?

(See Resources 14–1 and 14–2 for assistance in refining and completing the algorithm.) If the finished product passes this final test, it is time for the team to move on to Phase III, Implementation Strategy.

Resource 14–1

○ ○ ○ ○ ○

Algorithm Completion

Having completed the algorithm flowchart and the seed algorithm, the team begins to review and refine the algorithm. For this project to be successful, the algorithm must meet both patient and algorithm users' needs. Consequently, the team should review the information in Steps 6 and 8 and keep this information in mind as the algorithm is being completed.

HELPFUL HINTS

- After listing the patient needs from Step 6, the team determines whether this algorithm meets those needs.
- The team should follow the same procedure for the needs of the algorithm users, as found in Step 8.
- Any modifications or revisions that must be done should be discussed.
- It is easy for patient and algorithm user needs to get lost during the challenging beginning steps of algorithm development. Now is the time for the team to recognize any oversights and correct them in the final draft of the algorithm.

Resource 14–2

○ ○ ○ ○ ○

Algorithm Completion: Considerations

Algorithm Title

Date

1. List the patient needs identified in Step 6. Is each need met or not met by the algorithm?

   Need   *Met / Not met*

   _____   _____

   _____   _____

   _____   _____

   _____   _____

   How must the algorithm be modified so that all patients' needs can be met?

2. List the needs of the clinicians, as found in Step 8. Has the algorithm met/not met those needs?

   Need   *Met / Not met*

   _____   _____

   _____   _____

   _____   _____

   _____   _____

   How must the algorithm be modified so that all clinicians' needs can be met?

Phase IV

○ ○ ○ ○ ○

Implementation Strategy

The tasks of defining "best practice" and writing a clinical algorithm that results in every patient receiving optimal care are arduous indeed. The steps involved in the successful implementation of the algorithm may prove to be just as difficult. Often, this difficulty centers around the problems associated with gaining compliance. Thus, it is essential to have a plan of action to implement the algorithm and to have a system in place to ensure compliance by all clinicians.

In the United States, clinicians have a history of very poor compliance with medical algorithms. The health care changes in the next decade will require clinicians and medical organizations to define best practice for their particular situations and to standardize their clinical activities. By so doing, clinicians will strengthen their positions with third-party payers and increase their share in an ever constricting marketplace.

Step 15

○ ○ ○ ○ ○

Develop "Compliance Systems" for Algorithm

Develop
"compliance
systems" for
algorithm users

15

A compliance system is a planned approach to give compliance and support to algorithm users at crucial steps in the clinical process. The successful implementation of such a system ensures that the agreed upon "best practice" is provided to all patients.

With the introduction of any algorithm or new treatment activity, there is a wide range of acceptance among clinicians. Attitudes may fall along a compliance continuum as follows:

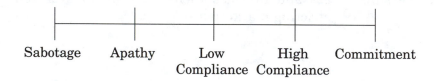

Sabotage   Apathy   Low   High   Commitment
                    Compliance   Compliance

In order to move all clinicians to the right in this continuum, the algorithm team should develop a plan to encourage high compliance and commitment among clinicians. Some algorithm users may be in the commitment range as soon as the algorithm is introduced. More likely, however, clinicians will move up the commitment continuum as they begin to experience the quantitative evidence of standardizing clinical processes. This is the reason for developing algorithms within an organization—to provide just such clinical evidence. For example, patients might be getting better in a shorter time, fewer tests are needed to diagnose the problem, shorter turnaround time needed for lab results, or patient satisfaction may be improving with the services provided (See Resources 15–1 and 15–2 for assessing clinician compliance.)

Algorithm compliance systems can be categorized simply as (1) those currently in place (often formal structures mandated by the organization) and (2) those newly developed by the algorithm team. The team first evaluates the compliance structures already in place within the organization, such as policy/procedures manuals, orientation sessions, peer review, in-service training sessions, coaching/mentoring sessions, and quality assurance activities. All these structures, no doubt, emphasize the importance of algorithm compliance, but they will probably not be enough to ensure compliance by the clinicians. The team must devise methods to give the clinicians the skills, tools, and education needed to comply with each step of the newly completed clinical algorithm.

To develop an effective compliance system, the team must look at each step in the algorithm to determine the places where compliance can be ensured. This is often a very difficult discussion for clinicians, and the facilitator must encourage all team members to be creative. Each member must realize that this is the make-or-break point in this long process.

> The reason most medical algorithms fail is that there is no support system developed to ensure compliance on a day-to-day basis.

James[1] discusses one method used to gain physician compliance. According to James, a major reason that a physician might demonstrate low compliance with an algorithm is the issue of "control." Clinicians view organization-mandated guidelines as mechanisms for administrators to restrict clinical judgment and control costs.

James describes how one team regained a sense of control over a clinical guideline that was being implemented in a large hospital. The clinical team was given a guideline for treatment of a particular clinical activity. The guidelines were very specific and were posted in the patients' charts as well as at the bedsides. As with most guidelines, the clinicians were expected to comply. However, it was made clear from the start that if a clinician's judgment caused him or her not to follow the guideline, it was assumed that the guideline was incorrect for that particular decision. Therefore, instead of blaming or reprimanding the clinician for failing to follow the guideline, the team looked upon these instances as opportunities to improve the guideline.

At weekly staff meetings, all instances of deviation were reviewed and the team decided if the guideline was correct, incorrect, or if a patient was an "outlier" for a clinical decision. According to James, one cannot expect a document structured as a guideline or algorithm to cover all patient variants.

By placing trust in the clinical skills of the team members (and not in the untested clinical guideline), the organization gave the

NOTES

team control over the clinical activity. As the guidelines were challenged, reviewed, and revised (if necessary) at weekly meetings, compliance by the clinicians markedly improved. In the brief span of four months, the percentage of total protocol instructions followed increased from 40 to 90 percent.

A tool often used in developing a compliance system for an algorithm is a fishbone diagram. This is a popular problem-solving technique that requires the users to organize potential causes of a problem into major categories: people, methods/documentation, materials, equipment, and miscellaneous. This type of diagram was introduced in the 1950s by Dr. Kaoru Ishikawa.[2] Its purpose is to ensure that all possible causes are considered when examining a particular problem. Constructing one clearly demonstrates where the name came from—it looks like a fish skeleton when completed. Usually, the diagram runs from left to right, with the problem statement in the box at the extreme right. However, the team can also use a backward fishbone diagram. The structure is similar, but now the goal of algorithm compliance is placed in the box on the left side of the diagram. This simple change in the structure of the diagram changes the way people view it. Instead of looking at possible problems that would prevent something from happening, the team looks at potential solutions that would ensure the algorithm's success. The same major headings are used, but the focus of the group is now on the positive. The question now becomes, what can we do to be sure that all clinicians will use this algorithm at every step in the treatment process? (See Resources 15–3 through 15–6 for developing fishbone diagrams.)

(*text continued on p. 97*)

NOTES

Resource 15–1

○ ○ ○ ○ ○

Clinician Compliance Assessment

As the algorithm team progresses through all the steps of algorithm development, it will become apparent that there is going to be some resistance on the part of clinicians who will be using the algorithm. With an understanding of what this resistance may entail, the team can reduce resistance and assist clinicians in changing their clinical practices with the least amount of fear, "pain," and/or intimidation.

The purpose of this information is for the team to understand the underlying causes of resistance and prepare the team to develop "process reminder systems" in the next steps.

HELPFUL HINTS

- Each member should fill out a copy of Resource 15–2. The facilitator can record the responses on a chartboard and can lead the team in a discussion of "key insights."

- Questions 1a and 1b will help the team understand the size of the gap between the compliance level that is likely now and the compliance level that is needed in 12 months.

- After the team identifies possible noncompliant behavior, the facilitator should lead a discussion of the underlying reasons for such noncompliance.

- The most valuable aspect of this exercise is the listing of the "key insights" regarding any behavior that can be viewed as resistance to the algorithm. This understanding will help the team in the development of "process compliance systems" in the next steps.

- If desired, Resource 15–2 can be modified and used as a survey of the clinicians who will be using the algorithm.

Resource 15–2

○ ○ ○ ○ ○

Clinician Compliance Assessment: Evaluation Form

_____   _____
Algorithm Title   **Date**

1. Rank your colleagues' likely response to this new algorithm.

   a. Mark on the continuum where compliance is likely to be when algorithm is first enacted.

   b. Mark on the continuum where it needs to be in a year to succeed.

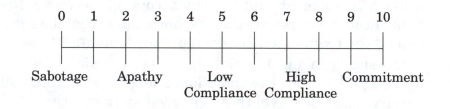

   c. Describe why you marked the continuum as you did.

   _____

   _____

   _____

   _____

2. List possible clinician behaviors that could be evidence of different levels of compliance.

   a. Understanding the resistance:

   _____

   _____

   1) Examples of "sabotage" behaviors _____

   _____

    2) Examples of "apathy" behaviors _____

_____

    3) Examples of "low compliance" behaviors _____

_____

  b. Understanding "Supportive" Behaviors:

_____

    1) Examples of "high-compliance" behaviors _____

_____

    2) Examples of "commitment" behaviors _____

_____

Resource 15–3

○ ○ ○ ○ ○

Using the Fishbone Diagram in Developing Compliance Systems

At this point, the facilitator leads the team in an exercise to develop a fishbone (or cause-and-effect) diagram. It may be helpful for the team members to collect some brief data from their colleagues before the meeting. This can be done in a survey, informally on a one-to-one basis, or in the next staff meeting.

Team members should complete Resource 15–4 prior to beginning the fishbone diagram. After its construction, the team needs to prioritize the causes.

HELPFUL HINTS

- The team must agree on the "effect box" before completing the form and beginning the fishbone diagram.
- The "effect box" must be a negative statement, such as "all patients reporting to the ER with chest pain are not being scheduled for a treadmill test." If the statement is not negative, the items will subtly shift from causes to possible solutions.

Resource 15–4

○ ○ ○ ○ ○

Using the Fishbone Diagram in Developing Compliance Structures

_____   _____
Algorithm Title   **Date**

In preparation for the algorithm team developing a fishbone diagram, complete the following to understand key causes of noncompliance with the new algorithm. (Review Step 14 in text.)

1. List possible reasons/causes of noncompliance with the new algorithm relating to methods (i.e., work process or documentation).

   _____

   _____

   _____

   _____

2. List possible reasons/causes of noncompliance with the new algorithm relating to people.

   _____

   _____

   _____

   _____

3. List possible reasons/causes of noncompliance with the new algorithm relating to equipment.

   _____

   _____

   _____

   _____

4. List possible reasons/causes of noncompliance with the new algorithm relating to materials.

_____

_____

_____

_____

5. List possible reasons/causes of noncompliance with the new algorithm relating to miscellaneous issues.

_____

_____

_____

_____

Resource 15–5

○ ○ ○ ○ ○

Example of a Fishbone Diagram

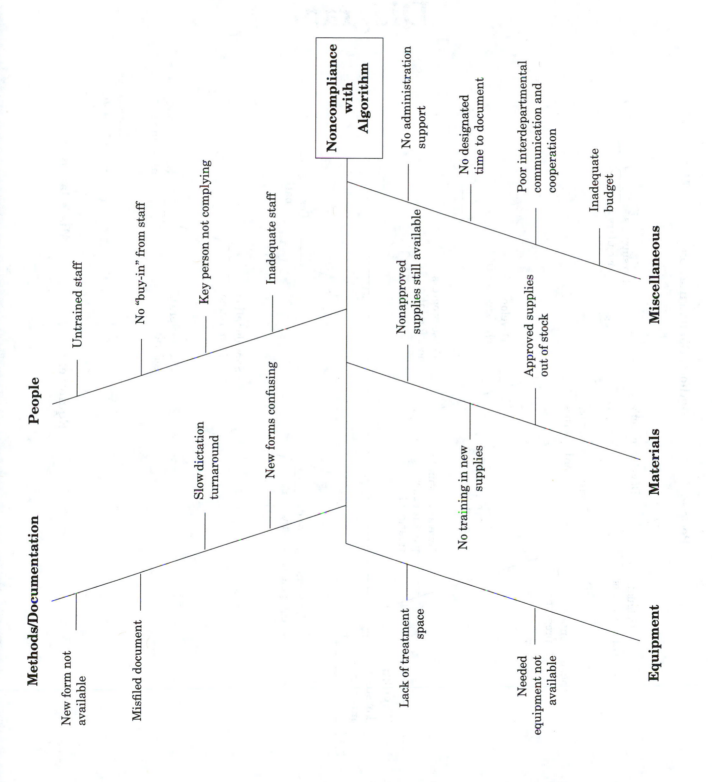

Resource 15–6

● ● ● ● ●

Example of a Backward Fishbone Diagram

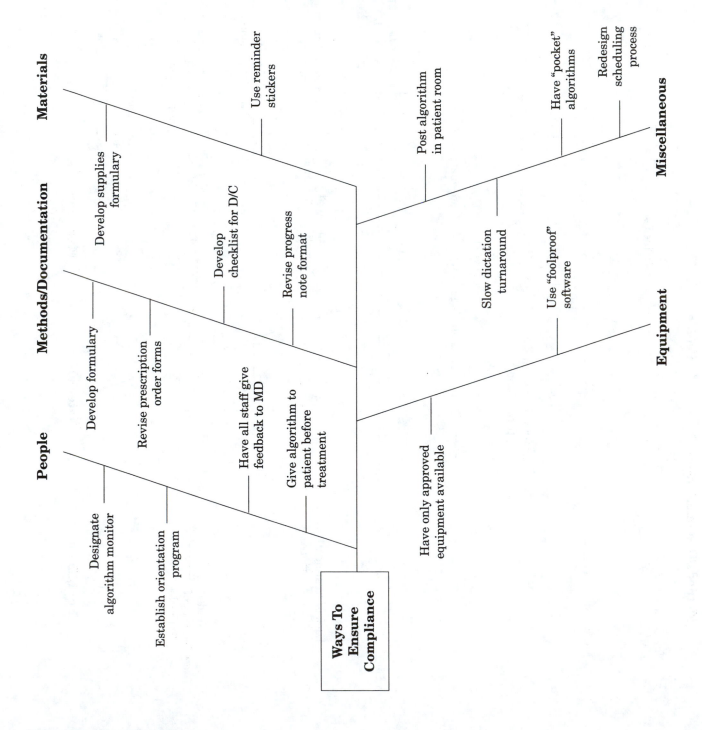

THE FOUR C'S

Once the diagram is complete and the team has considered all possible means of reminders, the facilitator needs to use *the four C's* involved in the prioritization of any list: **clarification, combination, criteria, and choices.** *Clarification* simply means that all team members understand each item. For all team members to participate in the prioritizing process, there must be no confusion about the meaning of each item. The facilitator then helps the team combine any two (or more) items that may be describing the same thing.

The third *C* is *criteria.* The team is asked, "What criteria will we use to determine which option is best for ensuring compliance in our situation?" Typical criteria include the cost of implementing the compliance system, the feasibility of the compliance system, solution, and the degree of impact that the compliance system will have on the organization. If any of the techniques are resource-intensive, it may be necessary to consult the steering group before taking further action.

Once the team members understand all the criteria to be used, it is time to make choices. Any number of methods can be used to vote on techniques to promote compliance, but the facilitator must try to avoid possible instances of "groupthink" that may occur when there are strong personalities involved.

The team has now selected a few techniques to implement for the algorithm reminder system. (See Resources 15–7 and 15–8 for assistance in constructing reminder systems. See Resources 15–9 and 15–10 for assistance in modifying present compliance structures.) Assignments are made so that actions on each item will be completed on a set schedule. One or more of the items may even require a pilot test, which the team will have to devise. Once all assignments are completed, the team will have successfully finished the development of a system that will ensure compliance at every step of the new algorithm.

REFERENCES

1. B.C. James. Implementing Practice Guidelines through Clinical Quality Improvement, *Frontiers of Health Service Management* 100(1)(1993): 3–37.
2. M. Daniel Sloan, *How To Lower Health Care Costs by Improving Health Care Quality* (Milwaukee, WI: ASQC Quality Press, 1994).

NOTES

Resource 15–7

○ ○ ○ ○ ○

Constructing Compliance Systems

Resource 15–8 is designed to assist the algorithm team in developing usable reminder systems. The purpose of such compliance systems is to ensure that the algorithm users follow the steps agreed upon in the algorithm. The easier it is for the clinicians to use the algorithm, the higher the compliance rate will be. As the compliance rate increases, the organization is able to achieve "best practice" and to increase patient satisfaction.

Parts 1 and 2 of Resource 15–8 are designed to assist the team in gathering information about the characteristics of useful compliance systems. After these forms are complete, the team can summarize its ideas of possible compliance systems in a reverse fishbone diagram as discussed in the text regarding Step 15.

HELPFUL HINTS

- Any of the forms can be filled out by the individual team members prior to the meeting or by the entire team during the meeting. Completing the forms prior to the meeting can speed up the meeting and can add to the depth of the discussion. It is always helpful to give individuals a moment or two to develop their own ideas before bringing the team together for brainstorming.
- Any time the team uses brainstorming, it is helpful to review the ground rules. The purpose is to generate a high quantity of ideas or thoughts. Although clarification of comments is acceptable, no critical comments or judgments are allowed.

Resource 15–8

○ ○ ○ ○ ○

Constructing Compliance Systems: Information Forms

Part 1

_____   _____
Algorithm Title   **Date**

List some everyday reminders to help us remember things to do (e.g., grocery list, note in shirt pocket, preflight checklist, forms, pocket calendars, instructions).

Examples of reminders I have used or seen with computers or automation: _____

_____

_____

Examples of reminders I have used or seen at work: _____

_____

_____

Examples of reminders I have used or seen in the military or at school: _____

_____

_____

Examples of reminders I have used or seen in household duties:

_____

_____

Examples of reminders I have used or seen in maintaining cars or other equipment: _____

_____

_____

Examples of reminders I have used or seen in other areas:

_____

_____

○ ○ ○ ○ ○

Part 2

_____

Algorithm Title   _____

Date

Developing "foolproof" compliance systems.

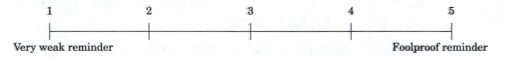

A foolproof reminder is defined as one in which the task cannot be completed unless the reminder system is followed (e.g., computer software that does not allow the user to proceed without completing certain steps.)

1. Based on the information developed on Part 1, list the reminders you identified which you believe would rank a 4 or 5.

   _____

   _____

   _____

2. List the characteristics of the foolproof reminders you identified. _____

   _____

   _____

3. List the points or steps in the algorithm at which these reminder systems are critical to ensure success of the algorithm.

   _____

   _____

   _____

4. Based on the characteristics of the robust foolproof reminders, list possible compliance systems to support the usage of the new algorithm, especially at the critical points. _____

   _____

   _____

Resource 15–8 <small>continued</small>

○ ○ ○ ○ ○

_____

Algorithm Title

_____

Date

Use the reverse fishbone to develop specific compliance systems (Resource 15–6, p. 96).

To assist the algorithm team in prioritizing the possible usable compliance reminder systems, complete the following for the information gained in Parts 1 and 2.

List possible compliance systems, structures, mechanisms, or activities in the area of **people supports** that would support the clinicians' use of the new algorithm. _____

_____

_____

_____

List possible compliance systems, structures, mechanisms, or activities in the area of **method and documentation supports** that would support the clinicians' use of the new algorithm.____

_____

_____

_____

List possible compliance systems, structures, mechanisms, or activities in the area of **machine or equipment supports** that would support the clinicians' use of the new algorithm. _____

_____

_____

_____

_____

Part 3 continued

List possible compliance systems, structures, mechanisms, or activities in the area of **materials supports** that would support the clinicians' use of the new algorithm. _____

_____

_____

_____

List possible compliance systems, structures, mechanisms, or activities in the area of **other/miscellaneous supports** that would support the clinicians' use of the new algorithm. _____

_____

_____

_____

Resource 15–8 continued

○ ○ ○ ○ ○

_____

Part 4

Algorithm Title

_____

Date

Determining action steps to develop key compliance systems.

1. List the required materials needed to develop the compliance system. _____

_____

2. List the actions needed to develop mock compliance system.

_____

_____

3. List the methods to test compliance system(s).

_____

_____

4. List possible costs of developing compliance system. _____

_____

5. List methods needed to train or orient algorithm users to compliance systems. _____

_____

6. Determine methods to measure success of compliance system.

_____

_____

7. Determine if any approvals are needed for compliance system.

_____

_____

8. Determine if reminder will complement similar compliance systems in related processes._____

_____

_____

Resource 15–9

○ ○ ○ ○ ○

Modifying Formal Organization Compliance Structures To Support the New Algorithm

The purpose of Resource 15–10 is to assist the algorithm development team in understanding and modifying the current organizational structures, policies, and practices to support the use of the algorithm. It is helpful to obtain assistance from administration, human resources department, and medical staff in determining the relevant organizational structures already in place.

HELPFUL HINTS

- One of the most influential forces within an organization to support change is the leadership, particularly at the senior level. The team should obtain feedback from personnel at this level concerning which leaders could provide visible, high-impact support for the algorithm.

- The team should also explore how the current "politics" of the organization might support or hinder the implementation of (and compliance with) the algorithm. The team should not hesitate to solicit the support of the steering group or the senior quality council.

Resource 15–10

○ ○ ○ ○ ○

Modifying Formal Organization Compliance Structures To Support the New Algorithm: Considerations

Algorithm Title _____ **Date** _____

1. List the current organizational policies, procedures, and practices that will or could support the utilization of the new algorithm (e.g., current or new policies, performance appraisals, supervisory structures, training or orientation programs).

   _____

   _____

   _____

2. List the current formal organization compliance structures that would have the greatest impact on ensuring the utilization of the new algorithm. _____

   _____

   _____

3. List ways that the current organization structures/policies need to be modified to support the new algorithm. _____

   _____

   _____

   _____

4. List the actions needed to modify current organization structures and policies. _____

   _____

   _____

5. Learn how senior management and leadership can and will support the compliance with the new algorithm.

   _____

   _____

   _____

Step 16

○ ○ ○ ○ ○

Assess/Address Organization Capabilities

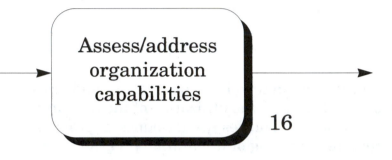

Assess/address organization capabilities

16

During Step 15, the team evaluated compliance systems designed to facilitate the implementation and accuracy of the algorithm. In Step 16, the team looks at organization-wide issues that may have a bearing on the successful implementation of the algorithm.

There may very well be systems or processes within the organization that, if not addressed, preclude the successful implementation of any algorithm. The algorithm development team attempts to identify those areas of possible algorithm breakdown and find ways to deal with them.

A cause-and-effect diagram is again useful to list all possible areas of concern. After all items are listed, the facilitator employs the *four C's* again—clarification, combination, criteria, and choice—and assigns action steps for the items chosen.

Representatives from other departments within the organization may be asked at this stage to take part in the discussion. The team may single out a person or group within the organization that is critical to the successful implementation of this algorithm. That person or a representative from that group must be present during the discussion of Step 16 so that all potential system breakdowns are identified and addressed. (See Resources 16–1 and 16–2 for assistance in assessing system capabilities.)

In the total knee replacement algorithm found in Appendix A, for example, the successful completion for Postoperative Day 1 requires communication and cooperation between several departments within the hospital. All of these departments are involved in the care of patients who have undergone this procedure. At least three other departments must carry out processes before the physical therapy department can successfully complete this algorithm. The dietary department must be consulted to establish when the patient will be finished eating. Nurses must have patients properly dressed, toileted, and medicated before rehabilitation services begin. Finally, both the physicians and nurses should begin rounds promptly at their scheduled time to facilitate patient treatments.

Resource 16–1

○ ○ ● ○ ○

Analysis of the Capabilities of Other Organizational Systems

An algorithm development team needs to view the organization as a whole and to examine the interaction of each system or process with all the others. This is especially true as the team attempts to determine how the new algorithm will interact with structures already in place.

Resource 16–2 helps the team consider the impact of the new algorithm on existing clinical processes throughout the organization. Obviously, the team is interested in obtaining support for the new algorithm. In addition, however, the team wants to foster support for the processes and systems already in place within the entire organization.

HELPFUL HINTS

- It is valuable to have personnel from other departments, processes, or systems within the organization join the team in a collaborative discussion of the changes involved in implementing the algorithm.

- The team members and any other personnel present must clearly state their needs. The team must describe what must happen for the algorithm to be successful. Other personnel must be able to discuss the impact of the algorithm on their department. Finally, there must be a determination of the specific actions each person must take to ensure the effectiveness of the algorithm.

- Everyone involved should participate in follow-up meetings or communications. It may be necessary to make minor changes and improvements in the algorithm as new learnings are gained concerning its impact on everyone within the organization.

- Discussions with other representatives of the organization should stay focused on the needs of each department or system. The discussions must result in a mutually satisfying method to meet the needs of everyone who will be affected by the algorithm.

Resource 16–2

○ ○ ○ ○ ○

Analysis of the Capabilities of Other Organizational Systems: Considerations

_____   _____

Algorithm Title   **Date**

List an organizational system (or work process) likely to be affected by the implementation of the algorithm: _____

_____

1. Describe how it would interact with the operation of the new algorithm.

   _____

   _____

2. Indicate whether the other system would support or hinder the effectiveness of the algorithm.

   _____

   _____

3. Suggest a method to determine whether the other system can support the requirements of the algorithm. (It may be helpful to list the requirement/needs of the algorithm in relation to the other system).

   _____

   _____

4. Determine actions to modify, change, or enhance the other organizational system in order to support the algorithm. Can the algorithm be easily modified to accommodate the other system?

   _____

   _____

(Complete for each key organizational system that interacts with the algorithm.)

Step 17

○ ○ ○ ○ ○

Develop Education/"Buy-In" Strategy

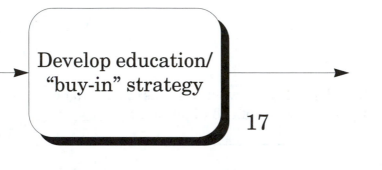

Develop education/
"buy-in" strategy

17

The team must identify the background, experience, and education that the algorithm users need to accept and comply with the clinical algorithm. Then, the team must develop a strategy to educate the algorithm users to gain their "buy-in." (See Resources 17–1 and 17–2 for assistance in developing an education strategy.)

Perhaps the most important method to gain buy-in by algorithm users is to educate, or train, all staff on the algorithm process. The team should determine the type of training that every person or group needs to use the algorithm successfully.

The team may be able to find other ways to gain compliance in the use of algorithms by brainstorming. Ideas can usually be divided into two categories: those that involve money and those that do not. Examples of ways to gain compliance include

- distribution of data on how algorithm compliance facilitates and/or improves patient outcomes
- distribution of data on algorithms as tools for market protection in the environment of health care reform
- illustration of algorithm's impact on the organization's financial performance (e.g., the number of procedures refused for payment by third-party payers)
- personal financial incentives
- clinic/department financial incentives
- peer recognition program
- supervisor reinforcement program

NOTES

Resource 17–1

○ ○ ○ ○ ○

Education Strategy for Algorithm Users

In developing an education strategy for algorithm users, the team should consider both teaching methodology and curriculum.

HELPFUL HINTS

- The team should first identify all groups that may be affected by the new algorithm.
- For each group affected by the algorithm, the team should identify the specific knowledge or skills needed to follow the algorithm. It is also necessary to decide who will be doing the instructing in these skills and what materials will be used.
- The skills of the algorithm users should be re-assessed following the training to ensure that all users have an understanding of any new procedures.
- The schedule of training must be realistic, considering the schedules of all clinicians involved.
- An educational specialist may be available from the human resources or medical education departments to assist with the training strategy and curriculum development.
- To facilitate "buy-in" by the users, it is often helpful to have a member of the algorithm team present for the additional instruction.

Resource 17–2

○ ○ ○ ○ ○

Education Strategy for Algorithm Users: Data Collection

_____   _____
Algorithm Title   **Date**

Education Needs of Associates

Associate	Areas of Additional Training	Who Trains?	How?	By When?
1.				
2.				
3.				
4.				
5.				
6.				
7.				
8.				
9.				
10.				

Step 18

○ ○ ○ ○ ○

Identify/Address User Concerns

```
┌─────────────────────┐
│                     │
│  Identify/address   │
│   user concerns     │
│                     │
│                 18  │
└─────────────────────┘
```

As stated earlier, the number 1 reason for algorithm failure is lack of user compliance. Thus, even though the team is composed of people who represent all algorithm users, it is important to take sufficient time to address needs and concerns of the people who will actually be using the algorithm. Every user should have a chance to meet with the team and discuss the implementation of the algorithm.

This meeting is potentially a time of heated discussion, resistance, and, possibly, even sabotage. If such trouble is anticipated, a member of the steering group can also attend to represent the administration.

The facilitator should make it clear at the outset that this is not the time to debate the pros and cons of the algorithm. The steering group has deemed the project necessary, and both the steering group and the algorithm development team have clearly stated the benefits of the algorithm. This meeting should identify user concerns and develop a plan of action to address those concerns. It should be clearly stated that the organization will offer any support and/or training deemed necessary to implement it successfully. (See Resources 18–1 through 18–3 for addressing algorithm users' concerns.)

At the end of this meeting the team may decide that a modification of the algorithm will make it easier to implement. This is an acceptable outcome of this meeting and will demonstrate that the team wants the algorithm to be "user-friendly."

NOTES

Resource 18–1

○ ○ ○ ○ ○

Addressing Algorithm Users' Concerns

It is a fundamental adage in the management of change that people support things they help to build. Realizing the truth of this statement, the algorithm development team involves the potential users of the new algorithm as much as possible. Resources 18–2 and 18–3 are designed to assist in gaining a "buy-in" on the part of all potential users. By addressing all the identified concerns of clinicians, the team demonstrates a commitment to creating "ownership"—both personal and professional—of the algorithm by all potential users.

HELPFUL HINTS

- Resource 18–2 can be used as a survey sent out to the potential users, or a sampling of such users can be invited to attend a portion of a team meeting. If a group setting is selected, each person should have the opportunity to voice concerns or comments; a vocal few cannot be allowed to dominate the discussion.

- Personal commitment increases in strength when an individual feels as if he or she has been heard. There must be time for everyone to share during the meeting.

- A lively discussion of viewpoints and a great deal of interaction helps to gain "buy-in." Conflict and disagreement are healthy aspects of this discussion. A lack of discussion may be an indication of low future compliance.

- Each participant in the meeting should be asked for his or her opinion on the algorithm and should be encouraged to support it.

Resource 18–2

○　○　○　○　○

Addressing Algorithm Users' Concerns: Questionnaire

_____   _____

Algorithm Title   **Date**

  The following questionnaire is designed to assist the algorithm development team in developing ways to support the effective use of this algorithm within the realities of clinical practice.

  The purpose and benefits of this algorithm are...(algorithm team to complete).

1. Initially, I envision the following barriers/obstacles in implementing this algorithm consistently in my practice: (Indicate with an asterisk * the primary barriers/obstacle.)

_____

_____

_____

_____

_____

2. What would help you in using this algorithm?

_____

_____

_____

_____

3. What are some of the potential benefits of the clinicians' consistent use of this algorithm?

_____

_____

_____

_____

4. What are some of the potential harms of the use of this algorithm?

_____

_____

_____

5. What are some of the personal/professional/clinical concerns that would prevent you from consistently using this algorithm?

_____

_____

_____

_____

6. What can be done to overcome these concerns in using this algorithm?

_____

_____

_____

_____

7. What are some possible ways to measure the effectiveness of using this algorithm?

_____

_____

_____

8. What can cause failure for this algorithm, and what can be done to prevent failure?

_____

_____

_____

Step 19

○ ○ ○ ○ ○

Plan Implementation of Algorithm

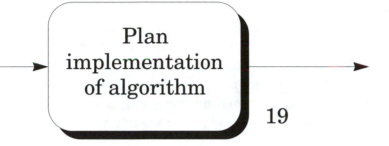

Plan
implementation
of algorithm

19

When all logistics have been identified and discussed, all accountabilities assigned, and all user concerns addressed, it is time to implement the algorithm. (See Resources 19–1 and 19–2 for implementing an algorithm.) A summary page such as the one shown in Resource 19–2 is used to assign accountability for each action deemed necessary to implement the algorithm. This page becomes the key document to track implementation. It lists the who, what, and when of every action being assigned.

The algorithm team should not get mired in efforts to estimate potential cost of implementing the newly developed algorithm. This is often a difficult and complex task, so the team should make its best effort and then move on. If necessary, the team can consult a person from the financial department for aid in making this estimate.

The successful completion of Steps 15 through 19 is cause for some celebration. Each of these steps is absolutely critical for the implementation of an algorithm that will help the organization standardize its clinical processes and face the challenges of health care in the twenty-first century.

NOTES

Resource 19–1

○ ○ ○ ○ ○

Algorithm Implementation Plan

It is essential to track the implementation of the overall algorithm development effort. The team, the leader, and the facilitator must be certain that all important actions are listed on a form such as Resource 19–2. This is an especially useful method to keep track of those steps that have yet to be completed.

One of the most common problems in algorithm development projects has been the lack of accountability for the actions that the team has decided to take. The team must devise a structured plan to assess continually the progress of the implementation. This plan should address what is working well, what still needs to be done, and who is going to perform the necessary tasks.

HELPFUL HINT

• A plan is essential to manage the change brought on by the implementation of this algorithm and to begin the application of the insights created by the algorithm.

Resource 19–2

○ ○ ○ ○ ○

Algorithm Implementation Plan: Summary

Algorithm Title   **Date**

Description	Required Action Steps	Person(s) Responsible	Month	Cost

INSTRUCTIONS FOR USE

1. **First column:** Complete the column with the major categories of actions such as system reminders, education of users, "buy-in" strategies.
2. **Second column:** List the actions for that major category.
3. **Third column:** Determine who will have primary accountability for the successful completion of each action step.
4. **Fourth column:** Estimate the completion date for this action step. Review the other steps that need to be taken, and be realistic with the estimate.
5. **Fifth column:** Attempt to estimate costs. These estimates will be useful to the senior quality council in its support of this algorithm.

Phase V

○ ○ ○ ○ ○

Monitoring and Evaluation

Once the algorithm is in place, the users are moving toward compliance with it, and they are beginning to learn from its use, it is essential to ensure that these learnings are used to build clinical knowledge in the department and throughout the organization. This short, but critical, phase of the algorithm development process is often referred to as "holding the gain." In other words, it is the task of the team to make sure that the benefits and learnings obtained from the use of the algorithm are continuously monitored, communicated to all interested parties, and used as stepping stones for further improvements. For a team to complete the algorithm development process without establishing a system to prevent the organization from regressing back to the "pre-algorithm" days would surely be a waste.

The organization has invested a great deal of time and resources in this project. During Phase V, the team has an obligation to develop a system that ensures a meaningful return on this investment.

Step 20

○ ○ ○ ○ ○

Determine Ongoing Measures

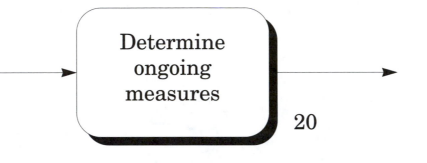

As discussed in Step 7, the algorithm team must ensure that there are reliable, quantitative measures in three categories:

1. patient satisfaction measures (e.g., percentage of patients in a particular diagnosis who were satisfied with their overall care)
2. clinical process performance measures (e.g., number of patients returning to surgery within 48 hours versus the total number of surgery patients)
3. clinical compliance and effectiveness measures (e.g., number of times the appropriate checklist was completed, number of times the appropriate test was ordered)

During Steps 11 and 12, the team developed specific clinical indicators to measure the effectiveness of the algorithm. Some of these indicators will now become part of an ongoing program to monitor the effectiveness of the algorithm.

To select the appropriate indicators, this team should review those listed during Step 12 and select the one or two that would be the most useful in monitoring the effectiveness of the algorithm for the first 6 months of use. This is a very important step—one that the algorithm team should not take lightly.

Monitoring of clinical indicators can be time- and resource-intensive for the person(s) responsible for the task. The team needs to prioritize the indicators and choose the one (ones)

NOTES

with the highest levels of reliability, specificity, validity, and sensitivity, as described during the discussion of Step 12. Such indicators make the task of monitoring easier and the data obtained of greater value to the team and the organization. (See Resources 20–1 and 20–2 for determining ongoing measures.)

The development of clinical indicators is a continuous, evolving process. Throughout the use of any algorithm, indicators are constantly modified and made more effective as the users gain knowledge from the use of the algorithm.

Resource 20–1

○ ○ ○ ○ ○

Determination of Ongoing Measures

One of the main purposes of developing a clinical algorithm is to create a structure that allows clinicians to apply new learnings and new knowledge. This structured approach, the scientific method, is based on a reliable and valid measurement system. For the algorithm, clinical indicators compose this system.

These measures enable the organization to refine and improve clinical processes continuously through learnings that are both reliable and valid. The measures themselves are also refined as the team gains insight into how the algorithm is actually working.

HELPFUL HINTS

- The expected clinical outcomes and clinical indicators developed earlier may be suitable for use as clinical process performance measures.
- The team needs to determine the criteria that will be used to assess such suitability. Such criteria may include ease of measurement, cost to the patient, and usefulness in future improvements.
- The team develops one or two key measures for each of the three categories of measures.
- It may be wise to seek assistance from departments within its organization, including financial planning.
- The essential component of a measure is that it provide useful clinical information for the purpose of improving the clinical practice.

Resource 20–2

○ ○ ○ ○ ○

Determination of Ongoing Measures: Considerations

Algorithm Title   **Date**

1. List the key patient satisfaction measures suitable for monitoring the impact of the new algorithm. (Prioritize one or two most useful measures.) _____

   _____

   _____

   Criteria used to identify key patient satisfaction measures...

   _____

   _____

2. List the key clinical process performance outcome measures suitable for monitoring the efficacy of the new algorithm. (Prioritize one or two of the most useful measures.) _____

   _____

   _____

   Criteria used to identify key clinical process performance outcome measures...

   _____

   _____

3. List the key clinical compliance measures to monitor essential aspects of clinical tasks outlined in the new algorithm. (Prioritize one or two most useful measures.) _____

   _____

   _____

   Criteria used to identify key clinical compliance measures...

   _____

   _____

Step 21

○ ○ ○ ○ ○

Develop Monitoring Methodology

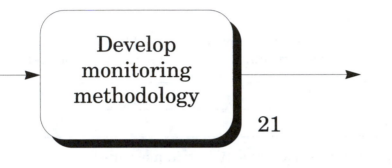

Develop
monitoring
methodology

21

To ensure accountability as to exactly who is going to monitor the use of the algorithm, the team must ask two questions: (1) Who is going to collect the data? and (2) Who is going to respond to any variances? An obvious third question follows: How is the team going to respond to any variances? A common cause of algorithm failure in an organization is uncertainty about who does what with the data collected. Reports produced by the algorithm monitor may be filed away and never see the light of day again.

After the team selects the person responsible for monitoring the clinical algorithm and the person responsible for responding to any variances, it must establish general guidelines to be used for reacting to any variances found in the data. (See Resources 21–1 and 21–2 for assistance in developing the monitoring methodology.) There is a general statistical guideline that the team can consider in reacting to variances in the data: All processes have natural variations that do not require a response. When the variations become trends or when unusual occurrences occur, the team is then obligated to investigate and respond.

A trend is generally defined as five consecutive points on a graph that go in one direction—either positive or negative. Such an occurrence warrants exploration into the possible reasons. It is acceptable for the team to use agreed upon limits of variation rather than statistical process controls. After these positive and negative limits of variation are in place, the team must investigate any indicator that goes beyond

NOTES

such limits. A special occurrence, such as the replacement of a vacationing employee with a temporary employee, may cause such a variation. In this case, the employee may not have received the training needed to complete the algorithm process successfully. To correct this situation, the team may decide to develop a "temporary employee survival kit" to educate all new personnel on what is expected of them.

When dealing with special occurrences that lead to variations, the team must remain aware that a single problem/situation is being isolated and addressed. It is not necessary to change the entire algorithm. In fact, changing the algorithm at this point would be "tampering" and would damage the credibility of the entire algorithm process. For clinical algorithms to be effective and accepted by clinicians, they must be based on scientific method and follow a step-by-step, logical approach to patient care. Any instances of tampering would put the success of the algorithm in jeopardy.

NOTES

Resource 21–1

○ ○ ○ ○ ○

Monitoring Methodology

A structure of accountability is necessary to ensure that the measurement system and the implementation of the algorithm are successful. The essential component of the measurement system is the production of useful information to continuously improve the clinical process being investigated. When all three sets of measures are utilized (i.e., patient satisfaction measures, clinical process outcome/performance measures, and clinical compliance measures), the satisfaction level of both the patient and the clinician increases.

HELPFUL HINTS

- Someone from the team should contact the supervisor of the person designated to collect the measurement data to be sure that he or she has adequate time and resources to fulfill additional responsibilities. It is also necessary to determine the appropriate format of the data collected.
- The team decides how often to collect data. A rule of thumb is to collect data at least once in every repeatable cycle of the process (e.g., daily, weekly, the first of every month).
- The team determines the threshold at which there will be a response in the algorithm process and the type of action that will be triggered.
- The team must have reliable and valid clinical compliance measures. If the process is unstable and has too many variables, there is no scientific way of understanding changes in patient outcome.

Resource 21–2

○ ○ ○ ○ ○

Development of Monitoring Methodology: Worksheet

Algorithm Title   **Date**

Key Measures	Who to Collect Data	How Often	Who Responds	At What Point (Threshold)	What Action Is Triggered
1. Patient Satisfaction Measures					
2. Clinical Process Performance/ Outcome Measures					
3. Clinical Compliance Measures					

Step 22

○ ○ ○ ○ ○

Develop Algorithm Follow-Up Plan and Identify Algorithm Process Owner

> Develop algorithm follow-up plan and identify algorithm process owner
>
> 22

Not only is it essential to provide structured accountability so that the expected outcomes of the algorithm can be achieved, but also it is critical to ensure that clinicians have access to new knowledge gained from the algorithm and are able to apply it. These goals require a follow-up plan. Usually, the team (or a committee designated by the team) is responsible for reviewing the entire algorithm effort. Before the algorithm is completed, this group should be identified and have answers for the following questions:

- When are we meeting again?
- What are we going to review?
- What indicators will we be reviewing?
- Who is to supply us with that data?

At the follow-up meeting, the group asks itself,

- What's working well in the algorithm?
- What needs to be addressed?
- Have there been any special occurrences that resulted in variations?
- Have any trends been established?
- Who is to address these and other issues that arise?

At this time, the team designates another important individual among its members—the algorithm process owner.

NOTES

This is the person who carries out the difficult (and sometimes thankless) job of monitoring the algorithm within the organization. The process owner assists in monitoring the indicators, follows through on any actions assigned, develops in-service training programs on the use of the algorithm, and performs any other task that facilitates the efficient use of the algorithm within the organization. At any follow-up meetings, the process owner is the person who provides updates as to what seems to be working and what is not. (See Resources 22–1 through 22–3 for information on the algorithm follow-up plan and identification of the algorithm process owner. See Resources 22–4 and 22–5 for information on the algorithm hand-off plan.)

NOTES

Resource 22–1

○ ○ ○ ○ ○

Algorithm Follow-Up Plan and Designation of Algorithm Process Owner

Resource 22–2 provides a format for the algorithm development team in determining the logistics of following up on the implementation plan. Resource 22–3 is the suggested agenda for the follow-up meeting, which can be conducted by the process owner with assistance from the facilitator.

HELPFUL HINTS

- The team completes Resource 22–2 as a group during the last algorithm development meeting before handing off the algorithm to the entire organization.
- Before the selection of a process owner, it is helpful to describe an effective process owner for this algorithm. The team should also determine to whom the process owner will be accountable.
- The agenda should be distributed prior to the meeting so that the team members can gather information and feedback from their colleagues.
- The follow-up meeting is a critical step in the ongoing improvement process. Without this follow-up and its clear accountabilities, the algorithm's long-term effect is likely to be diminished.

Resource 22–2

○ ○ ○ ○ ○

Development of Algorithm Follow-Up Plan and Identification of Algorithm Process Owner: Considerations

_____   _____

Algorithm Title   **Date**

The team completes the following:

1. When are we meeting again to review the implementation plan?

   _____

   _____

   _____

2. What are we going to review?

   _____

   _____

   _____

3. What indicators will we be reviewing?

   _____

   _____

   _____

4. Who is going to supply us with data?

   _____

5. Who is responsible for arranging the meeting, scheduling the room, and notifying the team?

   _____

   _____

Resource 22–3

○ ○ ○ ○ ○

Algorithm Follow-Up Meeting Agenda

_____   _____
Algorithm Title   **Date**

I. Purpose of the meeting

A. To gather learnings regarding the algorithm and its implementation efforts

B. To develop the next steps in understanding and improving the clinical activity being studied

II. Key learnings in each of the following areas

A. What is working well in the algorithm and the implementation?

B. Have there been any special occurrences?

C. Have any trends been observed?

D. What learnings have we gained from the algorithm's key measures (patient satisfaction, clinical process performance/outcome, and clinical compliance measures)?

E. How have the structures for the following worked?

1. the ongoing orientation/education of new clinicians regarding the algorithm

2. the monitoring methodology for the three sets of key measures

3. the effectiveness of the process owner role

III. Ongoing action plan for continuous improvement

A. Based on learnings and discussion, what are the key issues that need addressing?

B. Who will be responsible to address each issue and by when?

C. When will these actions be followed up and by whom?

Resource 22–4

○ ○ ○ ○ ○

Algorithm Hand-Off Plan

The purpose of a hand-off plan is to provide the essential organizational structures needed to achieve success for the algorithm and its users. The team completes Resource 22–5 and discusses it with members of the steering group, who have the authority to implement the final plan.

The steering group (or a representative) should attend one of the final team meetings for an update of the progress of the effort. A discussion off the hand-off options should be held, and the steering group should decide how and when any issues will be resolved.

HELPFUL HINTS

- The extent of involvement of the steering group depends upon the complexity of the hand-off plan and its potential impact on the organization's systems, structures, and resources.

- The team should address the amount of time, resources, and commitment required of the process owner. The steering group will have to approve any major changes in job descriptions or responsibilities.

Resource 22–5

○ ○ ○ ○ ○

Algorithm Hand-Off Plan: Considerations

Algorithm Title _____

Date _____

1. What new responsibilities created in this algorithm effort need to be completed after the algorithm development team disbands (i.e., data collection, educational and implementation tracking responsibilities)?

   A. _____
   B. _____
   C. _____
   D. _____
   E. _____
   F. _____
   G. _____

2. Who will be accountable for the completion of each of these new responsibilities?

   Responsibility A. _____
   Responsibility B. _____
   Responsibility C. _____
   Responsibility D. _____
   Responsibility E. _____
   Responsibility F. _____
   Responsibility G. _____

3. Are there other options as to who will be accountable for these new responsibilities? _____

4. Who is going to have overall responsibility for the successful implementation of the algorithm and to be the recognized spokesperson for the algorithm?

   _____
   _____

Step 23

○ ○ ○ ○ ○

Hand-Off for Continuous Improvement of Algorithm

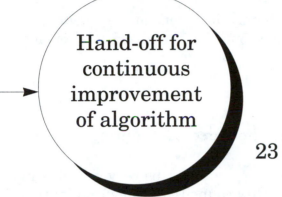

For most team members, the hand-off of the algorithm is a welcome relief after the long development process. With the completed algorithm, the team has set the stage for continuous improvement of patient care within the organization. The clinicians now have a structured method to build knowledge and to increase that knowledge base constantly.

The team and the steering committee must agree that the team has completed the algorithm development process and that the individuals concerned understand their specific assignments. It is of the utmost importance that the steering group (representing the organization) gives these individuals the resources they require for the successful use of the algorithm. (See Resources 23-1 and 23-2 for assistance in developing a plan to hand off for continuous improvement.) Additional topics of discussion involved in this step are likely to include the following:

- Who is to monitor the outcomes?
- Are outside experts to be used at any time?
- Who is to work with departments/individuals affected by this algorithm?

During this discussion, it is very important that clear accountability of resources is assigned and recorded. The more specific the assignments and the more clearly they are stated, the greater the likelihood that the algorithm will be successfully implemented.

NOTES

Resource 23–1

○ ○ ○ ○ ○

Hand-Off for Continuous Improvement

Resource 23–2 provides the team with a format to consider and address any final issues or "loose ends" in the algorithm development effort.

HELPFUL HINTS

- The team should complete Resource 23–2 during the final meeting.
- Feedback on the development process can be very valuable information for the senior quality council and the organization. Such feedback helps in the development of systems within the organization that will continuously improve clinical processes.
- An effective plan for communicating the successes of this project will help "sell" it and any future algorithms being considered.
- Part of the culture of continuous improvement is to recognize all members who have contributed to the development and success in a project. Even though the algorithm has yet to produce long-term results, the adage still holds: Recognize efforts and reward results. A final task of the team may be to create some kind of recognition event for its members.

Resource 23–2

○ ○ ○ ○ ○

Hand-Off for Continuous Improvement of Algorithm: Considerations

_____   _____

Algorithm Title   **Date**

1. What specific actions will the organization take to provide support for this algorithm?

   _____

   _____

   _____

2. Is there a mechanism in place for tracking the outcomes of this algorithm? Who passes the information on to the team? Who is to monitor the outcomes?

   _____

   _____

   _____

3. Are outside experts to be used at any time? (Who? For what? Who will contact them?)

   _____

   _____

4. Who is to work with departments/individuals affected by this algorithm?

   _____

5. Describe what worked well and what could be improved in this algorithm development process for future algorithm development teams? What have been the results to date regarding this algorithm effort?

   _____

   _____

6. Would it be helpful to communicate the efforts and results of this algorithm effort to others in the organization?

_____

_____

7. Are there final issues to address before handing off? Who is to document the algorithm team effort? How are the team members going to recognize and celebrate their efforts?

_____

_____

_____

_____

_____

_____

Phase VI

● ● ● ● ●

A Case History

The following case history illustrates the entire process of the development and implementation of a clinical algorithm. It also provides an opportunity for the authors to discuss trouble spots in the algorithm development process. Although the characters involved are fictional, there may be similarities between these characters and the experiences of the authors.

The utilization manager, Ms. Richards, of Pacific Goodhealth, a managed care organization in the Pacific Northwest, was reviewing the length of stay and the costs of treatment/rehabilitation associated with anterior cruciate ligament (ACL) surgeries in the last 2 years. Information obtained from health care purchasing cooperatives suggested to her that there was wide variation in the postoperative treatment of this type of surgery among orthopedists within Pacific Goodhealth. Through further research into the matter, Ms. Richards learned that there was no stable, standardized process for treatment of this type of patient within the organization.

Ms. Richards chose Evergreen Hospital, a community-based hospital with a strong orthopaedic practice to review the situation further. She discovered that, among the five orthopedists in a local group, there was also wide variation in the postoperative treatment of ACL patients. The senior quality council at Evergreen Hospital was notified of the variations and charged to investigate.

STEP 1: SELECT CLINICAL ALGORITHM

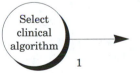

The senior quality council at Evergreen Hospital was composed of four members: (1) the hospital administrator, (2) the chief medical director, (3) the quality management director, and (4) the patient care administrator. As was the case in many smaller hospitals, Evergreen's senior quality council had appointed an ongoing steering group to oversee all hospital projects relating to clinical activities. The council appointed this steering group to oversee the ACL algorithm project.

The steering group was composed of five members: (1) chief of orthopedics, (2) chief of surgery, (3) chief of internal medicine, (4) medical director for quality management, and (5) the director of nursing services. Because Pacific Goodhealth had already suggested the clinical process to be studied, the steering group's next focus was on evaluating the potential impact of this algorithm on the day-to-day activities of the clinicians, patients, and third-party payers. After Dr. Moore, the quality management medical director, surveyed the appropriate personnel, it was determined that an ACL algorithm would have a significant positive impact on the organization.

Dr. Cummings, the chief of orthopedics, was asked to write a rough draft of a mission statement for the algorithm project. At a special meeting later that week, the steering group approved the final draft of the mission statement and turned its attention to selecting the members of the algorithm team.

STEP 2: SELECT ALGORITHM TEAM AND PROJECT LEADER

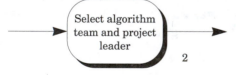

The steering group at Evergreen Hospital had a particular challenge in selecting the members of the algorithm team, because not all of the people directly involved with the postoperative care of ACL patients were hospital employees. Not only were the orthopedists in private practice across the street from the hospital, but also the primary physical therapy clinic was privately owned and operated. Because of the excellent professional relationship among the three entities, however, an effective algorithm team was selected. Its members were

1. Lawrence Archibald, MD, Orthopedics, Project Leader
2. Matthew Taylor, MD, Physiatry
3. Robert Kiley, PT, Outpatient Physical Therapy
4. Kirsten King, PT, Inpatient Physical Therapy
5. Jan Cunningham, RN, Orthopaedic Nurse
6. Olivia Olson, Facilitator

Because of his previous experience with quality improvement projects, Dr. Archibald was designated the project leader. Ms. Olson is an associate of the hospital in the quality management department.

Both Mr. Kiley and Ms. King are associates of Green Valley Physical Therapy, which operates the contract service with the hospital and a local outpatient therapy clinic. Dr. Taylor and Ms. Cunningham are hospital employees.

STEP 3: APPROVE ALGORITHM MSISSION STATEMENT

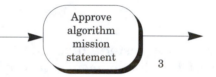

The Evergreen Hospital senior quality council officially approved the mission statement and the members of the algorithm team. In a memorandum to Dr. Archibald, the council expressed support for the project and assured him that Evergreen Hospital will provide the resources necessary to develop and implement the algorithm successfully.

Dr. Archibald and Ms. Olson met for the first time to discuss their individual responsibilities and duties. Because they had not had the opportunity to work with each other in the past, much of their first meeting was spent getting better acquainted. The remainder of the meeting was devoted to dividing various tasks between them and scheduling the first five or six team meetings. It quickly became apparent that seemingly simple tasks of scheduling meeting dates and times became difficult as the schedules of six people were involved.

After several attempts to accommodate all members of the team, the meeting dates were established and the team members notified of the first meeting in exactly 1 month. A brief summary of the issues that led to the algorithm effort was included in a packet sent to each team member.

STEP 4: HOLD START-UP TEAM MEETING

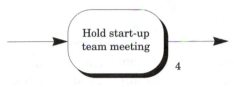

Both Ms. Richards and Dr. Moore were invited to attend the first meeting of the team to discuss the history of the questions involving the postoperative care of ACL patients. Ms. Richards strongly emphasized the need for stable, standardized clinical processes within the service districts of Pacific Goodhealth. Speaking on behalf of the steering group, Dr. Moore expressed support for the algorithm effort and pledged to make adequate resources available to the team to complete the project successfully.

Ms. Olson then led the team in a discussion of the algorithm process and its benefits to the organization, to clinicians, and to patients. Dr. Taylor expressed reservations about the algorithm process because of his previous experiences with algorithms when he was working for a managed care organization in Georgia. He noted that a great deal of time had been spent in creating an "official" document, but that no one had actually followed it. In addition, no one in the organization seemed to care enough to follow-up and determine if the algorithms were being used successfully. Despite these experiences, Dr. Taylor indicated a willingness to try again.

Ms. Olson reviewed the dates and times of the next five team meetings and asked if anyone had problems with any of the dates. Ms. Cunningham noted that her scheduled vacation conflicted with one of the meeting dates, and Mr. Kiley was scheduled to attend a continuing education course that conflicted with another. Those dates were changed, and the next five meetings were scheduled.

STEP 5: BRAINSTORM SYMPTOMS AND DRAFT/REVISE PROBLEM STATEMENT

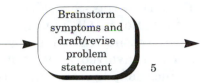

As the algorithm team began a brainstorming session, it became obvious that the members had very little understanding of their colleagues' interactions with the postoperative ACL patient. Ms. Cunningham did not know how the postoperative knee immobilizer was supposed to fit. Ms. King was not immediately aware of the requirements of the dietary department or of the nurses when dealing with a postoperative patient. Drs. Taylor and Archibald did not have the up-to-date knowledge concerning the appropriate rehabilitation exercises for the ACL patient. In other words, not every member of this team had a global perspective concerning the postoperative care of the ACL patient.

After this discussion, the team was able to draft a problem statement that accurately reflected the circumstances of the ACL patient at Evergreen Hospital:

> Currently, there is a wide variation in how we treat the postoperative ACL patient, resulting in longer periods of treatment, decreased patient satisfaction, and reduced reimbursement levels.

STEP 6: ASSESS PATIENT NEEDS

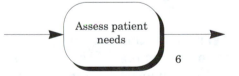

Like most health care facilities, Evergreen Hospital had conducted patient satisfaction surveys on a regular basis. Ms. King agreed to contact the patient relations department for information of value to the team. In addition, Ms. Olson led the team in an exercise designed to make the team members think like patients. Through this exercise, the team felt able to list the most pressing needs of the patient undergoing ACL surgery. With some mild reservations, it was decided that the team did not need to conduct any more formal surveys.

During this stage of the process, the team decided to slightly narrow the scope of the algorithm including only those ACL patients who underwent an ACL reconstruction using the patellar tendon of the involved knee. Notified of the slight modification, the steering group approved.

STEP 7: DEFINE EXPECTED OUTCOMES

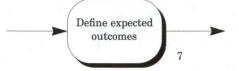

The mission statement that the senior quality council forwarded to the algorithm team contained expected outcomes that were, for the most part, appropriate. The outcomes were

1. increase in knee range of motion at 2 months postoperatively
2. decrease in the length of time in physical therapy following surgery
3. increase in patient satisfaction
4. decrease in the amount of time necessary for the patient to return to full activity
5. increase in the number of patients who received a functional brace for activities

STEP 8: ASSESS CLINICAL USER NEEDS

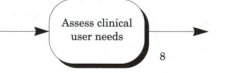

As may be expected, the algorithm team really struggled to get the rest of the clinicians to "buy into" the algorithm process. Dr. Archibald and Ms. Cunningham contacted the clinicians involved in the postoperative care of ACL patients to hear their need for this algorithm. One of the physicians noted that the algorithm had to incorporate the most up-to-date information concerning postoperative treatment of ACL patients; this physician felt that this is an area where the current rate of progress makes it difficult to keep up with the latest information. Other, more predictable

responses included, "Must be easy to use," "Must be cost-effective for the patient," and "Cannot add to paperwork."

STEP 9: REVIEW CURRENT PRACTICES AND IDENTIFY LEARNINGS

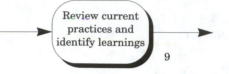

As the algorithm team reviewed current practices, the members gained some valuable information. The orthopedists had assumed that certain activities were taking place in physical therapy, and the physical therapists had assumed that the physicians were informing the patients of certain precautions. The review made it clear to everyone that these were incorrect assumptions and that there were huge communication gaps between the physicians and the therapy staff.

It was also discovered that different therapists were giving patients different information regarding the speed of recovery and return to full activities. There was also wide variation among the orthopedists, as Dr. Archibald treated his patients much more aggressively and encouraged them to resume normal activity earlier than did his associate, Dr. Armstrong.

After this enlightening discussion, Ms. Olson led the team in an effort to construct a flowchart that described the care given to the ACL patient after surgery.

STEP 10: REVIEW LITERATURE REGARDING "BEST PRACTICE" BASED ON RELIABLE RESEARCH

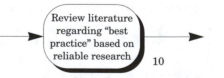

Dr. Taylor and Ms. King volunteered to conduct a search of the medical literature regarding the postoperative treatment of ACL patients. The team soon discovered that there is a plethora of articles in medical journals about ACL surgery. The members decided to limit their search to articles written in the last 5 years and to use only those articles that were written by one of five authors considered to be national experts (benchmarks) in the field. Even with these limitations, 23 articles were found and reviewed.

In a previous hospital position, Ms. King had worked with a recognized leader in the field, so she volunteered to contact that surgeon by telephone.

After gathering the pertinent information, the team members tried to decide which information was relevant for Evergreen Hospital. For example, two of the benchmark rehabilitation protocols recommended that the postoperative ACL patient begin walking in a swimming pool soon after the sutures are removed. As Evergreen Hospital did not have a pool and was not in a position to add a pool, this information was not included in the algorithm.

STEP 11: DEFINE CLINICAL OUTCOMES TO BE ACHIEVED

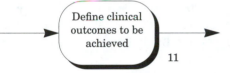

One of the most troublesome tasks for an algorithm development team is the definition of clinical outcomes. It took a great deal of patience on the part of Ms. Olson to lead the team through a discussion of the importance of quantifiable, valid outcomes. Examples of the clinical outcomes finally agreed upon are

- passive knee extension of 5 degrees or less at 2 weeks postoperatively
- hamstring strength 75% of that in the uninvolved leg at 6 weeks postoperatively

STEP 12: DEFINE POSSIBLE CLINICAL INDICATORS

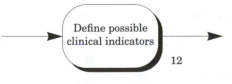

Even though every member of the algorithm team had a background in science and a famil-

iarity with the scientific method, it was difficult to develop clinical indicators. Ms. Cunningham obtained samples of clinical indicators that were included in the hospital's policy and procedure manual. After sometimes heated discussion, however, the team members decided that these were neither quantifiable, nor valid, indicators.

The following are two examples of clinical indicators adopted by the team:

$$\frac{\text{Number of ACL patients placed in the continuous passive motion device within 6 hours of surgery}}{\text{Number of ACL surgeries performed}}$$

$$\frac{\text{Number of ACL patients with 90 degrees of knee flexion at 1 week postoperative}}{\text{Number of ACL surgeries performed}}$$

STEP 13: IDENTIFY/DISCUSS SEED ALGORITHM

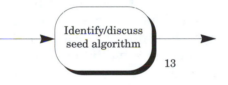

Somebody had to say it eventually, so Dr. Archibald immediately said, "Let's don't reinvent the wheel."

After the team members digested that bit of wisdom, Ms. Olson helped them to begin thinking about writing a seed algorithm for the treatment of ACL surgery patients. This is the point at which the team finally came to consensus about what constitutes "best practice" for the ACL patient at Evergreen Hospital. Although some of the more expensive equipment was not available to the physicians and therapists at Evergreen Hospital, the team was able to use the benchmark information to create its definition of best practice for patients who underwent ACL surgery at the hospital.

Because of the strong personalities involved in this group, it might have been helpful if one or two individuals had attempted to write the first draft of the seed algorithm before the entire team met to discuss the algorithm. Having everyone present to hash out every little step made the meetings longer and more stressful.

STEP 14: DEVELOP ALGORITHM USING STANDARDIZED FORMAT

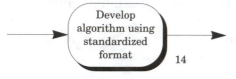

The expertise of Ms. Olson was evident throughout the algorithm development process, but her experience was nowhere more valuable than in the use of a standardized format for the algorithm. The team members quickly learned that there is a great deal of skill in creating an algorithm that does what it purports to do. The exact placement of symbols that represent tasks and questions is crucial to an effective algorithm.

Another demonstration of her considerable facilitating skills was the fact that Ms. Olson was able to bring Dr. Archibald and Mr. Kiley together on the important issues involved in ACL rehabilitation. These two strong-willed, intelligent people were able to reach consensus, and both expressed a willingness to "buy into" the completed document.

STEP 15: DEVELOP COMPLIANCE SYSTEM FOR ALGORITHM

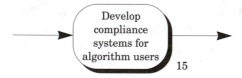

Recognizing the importance of commitment on the part of the algorithm users, the team spent a long session discussing ways to move all clinicians to the right on the compliance continuum. It was decided to encourage members of the outpatient rehabilitation group and the inpatient hospital department to establish their own ways to implement the algorithm and to report back to the group. One of the methods used by the inpatient team was a daily flowsheet that listed the expected outcomes for each patient every day. The outpatient therapists

devised a protocol in which measurable data determine the rate at which ACL patients progress.

Algorithm compliance systems already in place within Evergreen Hospital and Green Valley Physical Therapy included regular in-service training programs, coaching/mentoring sessions, policy/procedure manuals, regular team meetings, and regular physician/therapist meetings.

STEP 16: ASSESS/ADDRESS ORGANIZATION CAPABILITIES

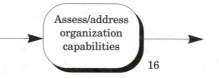

In examining individuals or issues within Evergreen Hospital that may preclude the successful implementation of this algorithm, the team decided that it was critical to gain "buy in" from Ms. Palance, RN, the shift supervisor in the recovery room. Ms. Cunningham was assigned to meet with her, to listen to her concerns, and to report back to the team by the next scheduled meeting.

Ms. King was to meet with a supervisor in the dietary department to work out a schedule so that the ACL patients would have eaten before they were supposed to begin physical therapy for the day. Finally, Mr. Kiley was to meet with the local pharmacist to ensure that both the postoperative knee immobilizers and the functional braces would be in stock and available when needed.

STEP 17: DEVELOP EDUCATION/"BUY-IN" STRATEGY

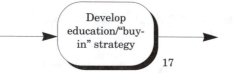

Each physician, staff, and physical therapy team scheduled in-service programs and educational meetings to discuss the workings of the new algorithm. Mr. Kiley and Ms. King were instrumental in organizing these meetings and leading the discussion concerning the benefits of the algorithm for all potential users.

Although the team discussed offering financial incentives to those who fully complied with the steps of the algorithm, it was decided to forego such incentives at this time.

STEP 18: IDENTIFY/ADDRESS USER CONCERNS

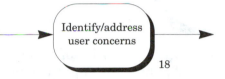

After using the new algorithm for a few weeks, the nursing staff at the orthopedist's office had some minor corrections and suggestions concerning the removal of the sutures and the settings on the knee immobilizer. The team addressed these suggestions at the next meeting and adjusted the algorithm accordingly.

It was at this meeting that a member of the inpatient physical therapy team, Jerry Schrader, PT, came to argue vehemently against the use of a document as "restricting" as an algorithm. Both Dr. Archibald and a representative from the steering group addressed Mr. Schrader's concerns, but both were firm in their commitment to the implementation of the ACL algorithm at Evergreen Hospital. Although Mr. Schrader was not entirely "sold," he was convinced that the hospital was willing to provide appropriate support and/or training to all staff. Perhaps more important, the team felt that he was moving in the right direction along the commitment continuum.

STEP 19: PLAN IMPLEMENTATION OF ALGORITHM

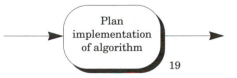

Ms. Olson had developed an assignment sheet and brought it to the team meeting. Every task that involved a who, what, and/or

when was recorded on the sheet. For example, Ms. Cunningham and Ms. King were to conduct an orientation meeting with the recovery room nurses by a certain date. Likewise, Mr. Kiley was to develop a monitoring system for the use of the continuous passive motion device.

STEP 20: DETERMINE ONGOING MEASURES

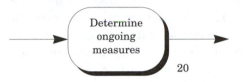

During the discussion of appropriate ongoing measures, the algorithm team re-examined the measures that had been discussed during Step 7. Because of the time and resources involved in obtaining such data, the team decided to focus on the "vital few" that would demonstrate the effectiveness of the algorithm. Following are the three that were chosen:

1. number of times the inpatient flowsheets were completed
2. passive knee range of motion at 3 weeks postoperatively
3. functional scale rating at 4 weeks postoperatively

There was much discussion about which measure would be the most helpful. The meeting ended with all members agreeing that it would be necessary to monitor, reconsider, and, quite possibly, revise the measures in the next months. Ms. King correctly pointed out that as knowledge is gained, the team will be expected to refine the measures to make them more exact.

STEP 21: DEVELOP MONITORING METHODOLOGY

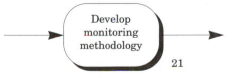

Mr. Kiley volunteered to head up a task group to monitor the algorithm. With assistance from an instructor at a local community college, the task force gained an understanding of statistical process controls. This knowledge enabled the task force to deal with a special occurrence (i.e., a new orthopedist's joining the practice) and to discover a trend in the passive range of motion of the postoperative knee. It seems that patients of the new physician were experiencing more difficulty in achieving complete range of motion of the knee. When the trend became clear, Mr. Kiley called a meeting of the algorithm team. After discussion and feedback from all clinicians, the use of the knee immobilizer was slightly modified.

STEP 22: DEVELOP ALGORITHM FOLLOW-UP PLAN AND IDENTIFY ALGORITHM PROCESS OWNER

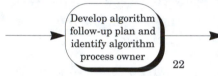

Mr. Kiley's task force was asked to review the entire algorithm effort. The group met monthly to look at the indicators and measures. With some hesitation, Dr. Taylor volunteered to be the algorithm process owner. Together with Dr. Archibald, Ms. King, and Mr. Kiley, he devel-

oped mechanisms to obtain the necessary information and share it within the hospital.

STEP 23: HAND OFF FOR CONTINUOUS IMPROVEMENT

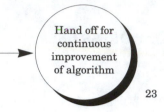

After approximately 11 months of meeting, discussing (arguing?), and planning, the development team handed off the ACL algorithm to the steering group of Evergreen Hospital. The mechanisms for tracking the effectiveness of the algorithm were reviewed. The members of Dr. Taylor and Mr. Kiley's task force were identified as the individuals responsible for tracking and reviewing the algorithm.

On behalf of Evergreen Hospital, the steering group expressed its appreciation to the algorithm development team and accepted the completed algorithm. At this meeting, the team made several recommendations to the steering group: monthly meetings for the task force, the limited use of a consultant in statistics, the development of new chart forms, and the purchase of two CPMs for the recovery room.

Appendix A

○ ○ ○ ○ ○

Total Knee Replacement Algorithm

Note:

Abbreviations used in Appendix A:

AAROM—active assistive range of motion
CPM—continuous range of motion device
EOB—edge of bed
ISLR—independent straight leg raise
mvmt—movement
PROM—passive range of motion
P.T.—Physical Therapist
PWB—partial weight bearing
ROM—range of motion
SBA—standby assist
TKR POD 1—Total Knee Replacement, Postoperative Day Number 1
TWB—Touch Weight bearing

Source: Courtesy of Black Hills Physical Therapy. © BHPT Corporation 1993. All Rights Reserved.

CLINICAL GUIDELINE DEVELOPMENT
Aspen Publishers, Inc.

Total Knee Rehabilitation
Day of Surgery

Expected outcome for the day:

1. CPM 0°–60°

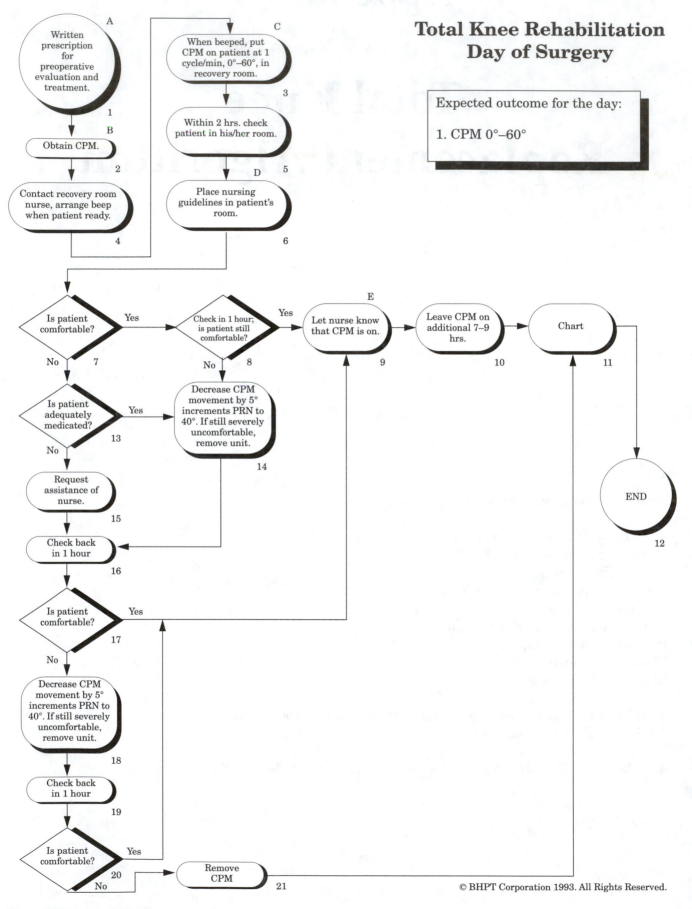

A
Written prescription for preoperative evaluation and treatment. — 1

B
Obtain CPM. — 2

Contact recovery room nurse, arrange beep when patient ready. — 4

C
When beeped, put CPM on patient at 1 cycle/min, 0°–60°, in recovery room. — 3

Within 2 hrs. check patient in his/her room. — 5

D
Place nursing guidelines in patient's room. — 6

Is patient comfortable? — 7
- Yes →
- No ↓

Check in 1 hour; is patient still comfortable? — 8
- Yes →
- No ↓

E
Let nurse know that CPM is on. — 9

Leave CPM on additional 7–9 hrs. — 10

Chart — 11

END — 12

Is patient adequately medicated? — 13
- Yes →
- No ↓

Decrease CPM movement by 5° increments PRN to 40°. If still severely uncomfortable, remove unit. — 14

Request assistance of nurse. — 15

Check back in 1 hour — 16

Is patient comfortable? — 17
- Yes →
- No ↓

Decrease CPM movement by 5° increments PRN to 40°. If still severely uncomfortable, remove unit. — 18

Check back in 1 hour — 19

Is patient comfortable? — 20
- Yes →
- No

Remove CPM — 21

Total Knee Rehabilitation Postoperative Day 1

Expected outcomes for today:

1. CPM 0°–60° 8–10 hours
2. Transfers with moderate assistance
3. Ability to stand at edge of bed 2–3 minutes TWB

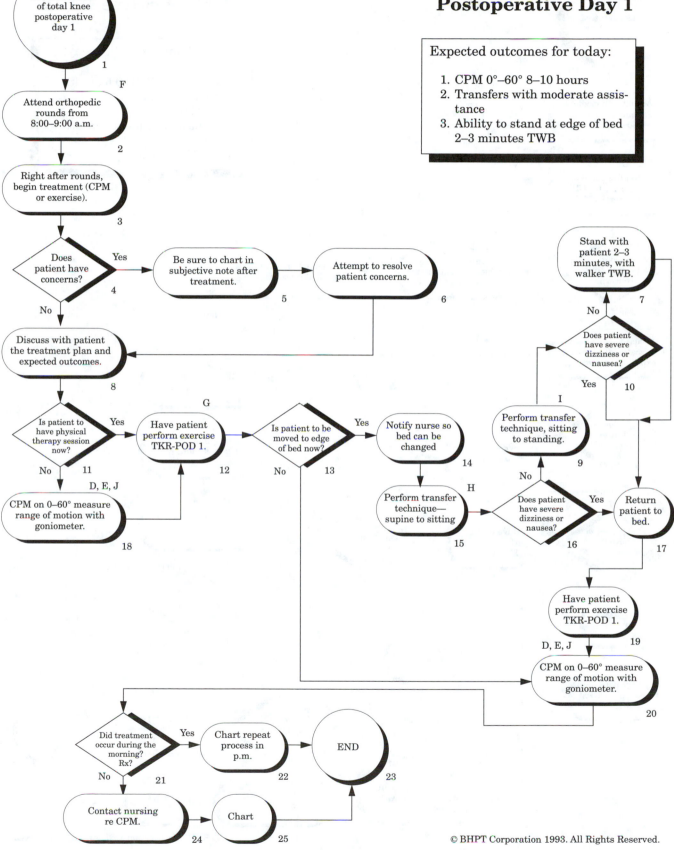

CLINICAL GUIDELINE DEVELOPMENT
Aspen Publishers, Inc.

Total Knee Rehabilitation
Postoperative Day 2

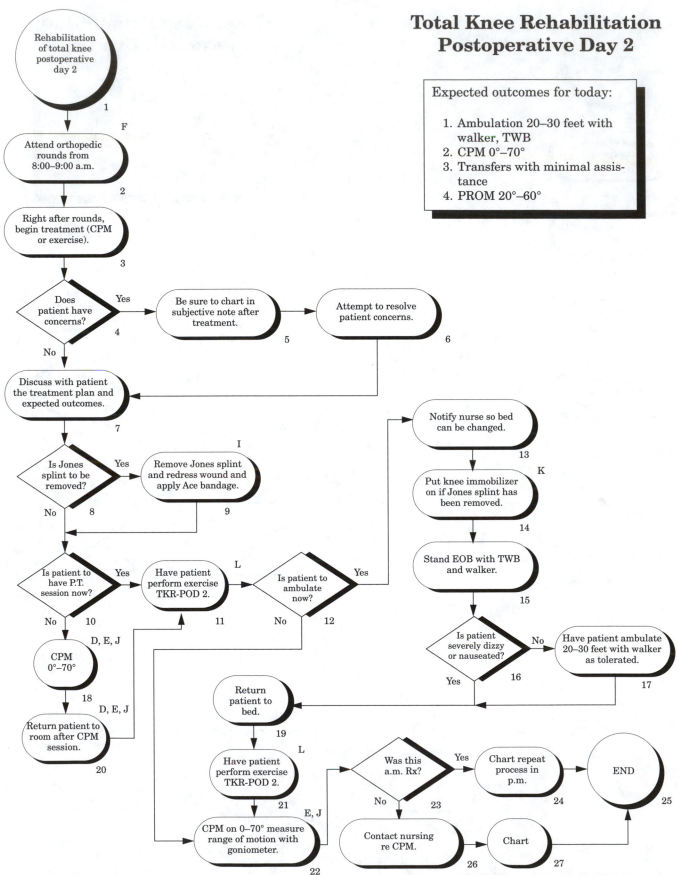

Expected outcomes for today:

1. Ambulation 20–30 feet with walker, TWB
2. CPM 0°–70°
3. Transfers with minimal assistance
4. PROM 20°–60°

1 Rehabilitation of total knee postoperative day 2

F

2 Attend orthopedic rounds from 8:00–9:00 a.m.

3 Right after rounds, begin treatment (CPM or exercise).

4 Does patient have concerns?
— Yes → 5 Be sure to chart in subjective note after treatment. → 6 Attempt to resolve patient concerns.
— No

7 Discuss with patient the treatment plan and expected outcomes.

8 Is Jones splint to be removed?
— Yes → I — 9 Remove Jones splint and redress wound and apply Ace bandage.
— No

10 Is patient to have P.T. session now?
— Yes → 11 Have patient perform exercise TKR-POD 2. → L — 12 Is patient to ambulate now?
— No → D, E, J

18 CPM 0°–70°
D, E, J
20 Return patient to room after CPM session.

12 Is patient to ambulate now?
— Yes → 13 Notify nurse so bed can be changed.
— No → 19 Return patient to bed.

K
14 Put knee immobilizer on if Jones splint has been removed.

15 Stand EOB with TWB and walker.

16 Is patient severely dizzy or nauseated?
— No → 17 Have patient ambulate 20–30 feet with walker as tolerated.
— Yes → 19 Return patient to bed.

19 Return patient to bed.

L
21 Have patient perform exercise TKR-POD 2.

22 CPM on 0–70° measure range of motion with goniometer.
E, J

23 Was this a.m. Rx?
— Yes → 24 Chart repeat process in p.m. → 25 END
— No → 26 Contact nursing re CPM. → 27 Chart → 25 END

Total Knee Rehabilitation Postoperative Day 3

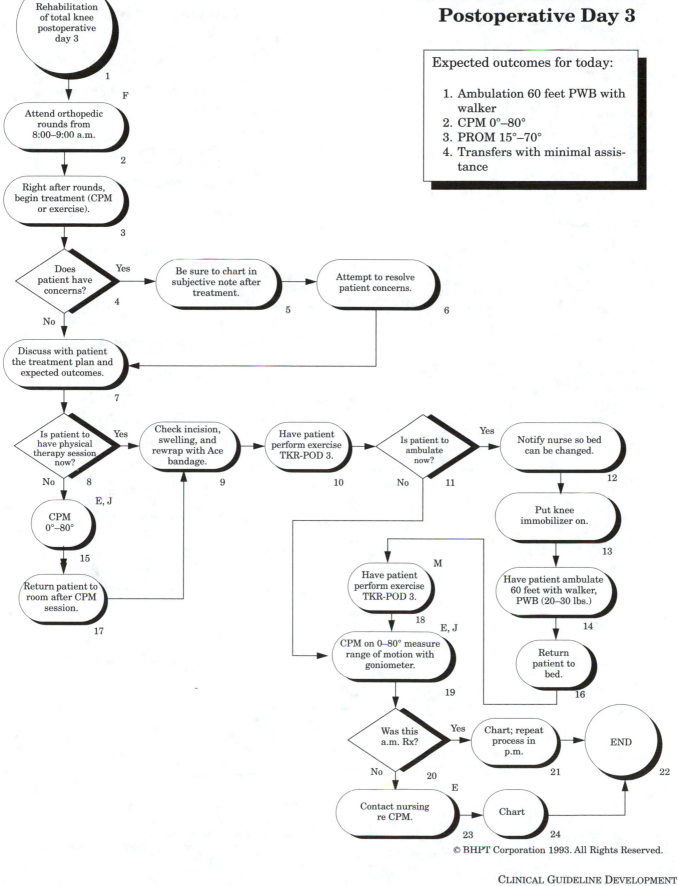

Expected outcomes for today:

1. Ambulation 60 feet PWB with walker
2. CPM 0°–80°
3. PROM 15°–70°
4. Transfers with minimal assistance

---

1 Rehabilitation of total knee postoperative day 3

F

2 Attend orthopedic rounds from 8:00–9:00 a.m.

3 Right after rounds, begin treatment (CPM or exercise).

4 Does patient have concerns?
— Yes → **5** Be sure to chart in subjective note after treatment. → **6** Attempt to resolve patient concerns.
— No →

7 Discuss with patient the treatment plan and expected outcomes.

8 Is patient to have physical therapy session now?
— Yes → **9** Check incision, swelling, and rewrap with Ace bandage. → **10** Have patient perform exercise TKR-POD 3. → **11** Is patient to ambulate now?
— No →

E, J

11 Is patient to ambulate now?
— Yes → **12** Notify nurse so bed can be changed. → **13** Put knee immobilizer on. → **14** Have patient ambulate 60 feet with walker, PWB (20–30 lbs.) → **16** Return patient to bed.
— No →

M

18 Have patient perform exercise TKR-POD 3.

E, J

19 CPM on 0–80° measure range of motion with goniometer.

15 CPM 0°–80°

17 Return patient to room after CPM session.

20 Was this a.m. Rx?
— Yes → **21** Chart; repeat process in p.m. → **22** END
— No →

E

23 Contact nursing re CPM. → **24** Chart → **22** END

CLINICAL GUIDELINE DEVELOPMENT
Aspen Publishers, Inc.

Total Knee Rehabilitation Postoperative Day 4

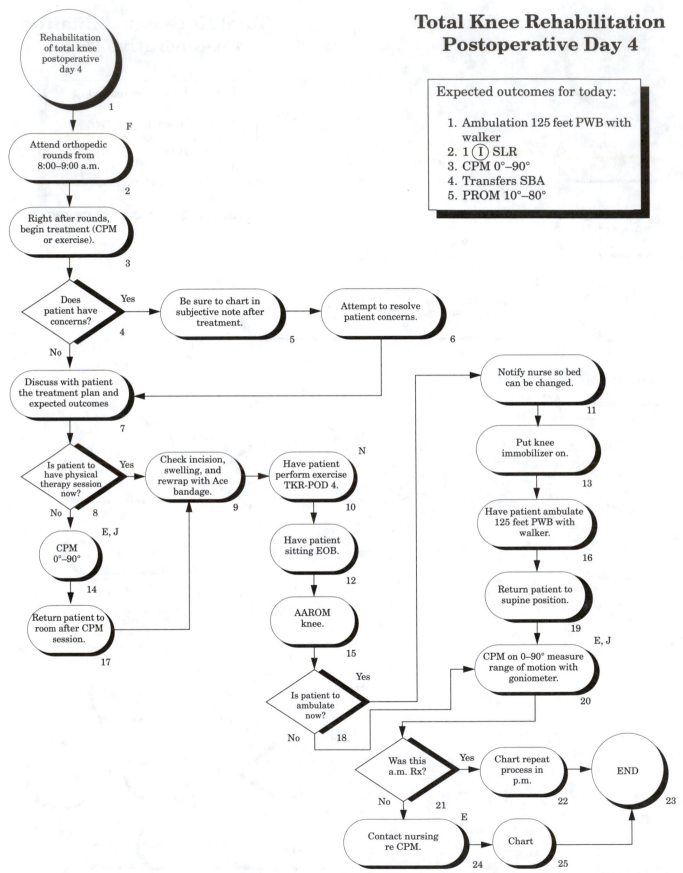

Expected outcomes for today:

1. Ambulation 125 feet PWB with walker
2. 1 (I) SLR
3. CPM 0°–90°
4. Transfers SBA
5. PROM 10°–80°

1. Rehabilitation of total knee postoperative day 4

2. Attend orthopedic rounds from 8:00–9:00 a.m.   F

3. Right after rounds, begin treatment (CPM or exercise).

4. Does patient have concerns? — Yes → 5. Be sure to chart in subjective note after treatment. → 6. Attempt to resolve patient concerns.

No

7. Discuss with patient the treatment plan and expected outcomes

8. Is patient to have physical therapy session now? — Yes → 9. Check incision, swelling, and rewrap with Ace bandage. → 10. Have patient perform exercise TKR-POD 4.   N

No   E, J

14. CPM 0°–90°

17. Return patient to room after CPM session.

12. Have patient sitting EOB.

15. AAROM knee.

18. Is patient to ambulate now? — Yes → 20. CPM on 0–90° measure range of motion with goniometer.   E, J

No

11. Notify nurse so bed can be changed.

13. Put knee immobilizer on.

16. Have patient ambulate 125 feet PWB with walker.

19. Return patient to supine position.

20. CPM on 0–90° measure range of motion with goniometer.   E, J

21. Was this a.m. Rx? — Yes → 22. Chart repeat process in p.m. → 23. END

No   E

24. Contact nursing re CPM. → 25. Chart

Total Knee Rehabilitation
Postoperative Day 5 to Discharge

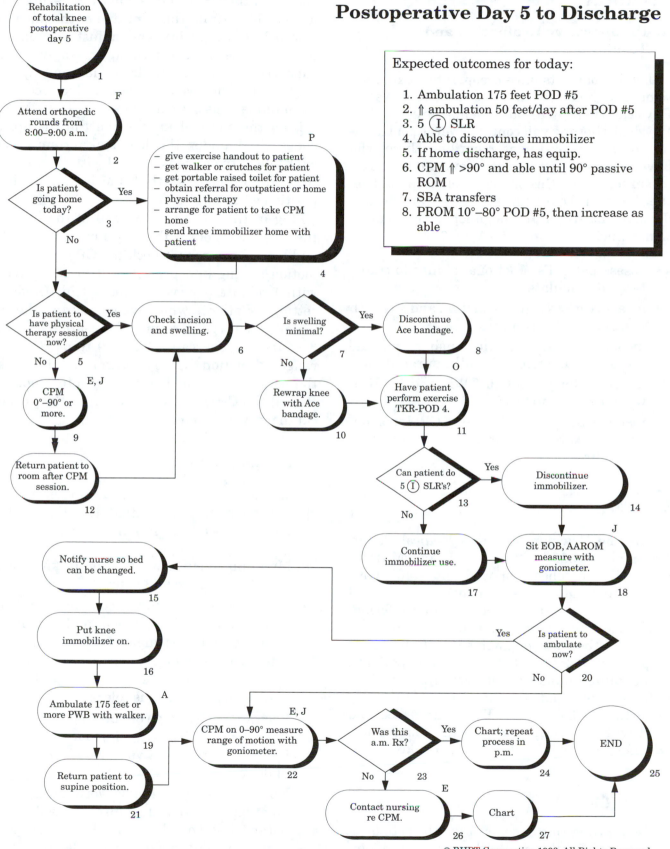

Expected outcomes for today:

1. Ambulation 175 feet POD #5
2. ⇑ ambulation 50 feet/day after POD #5
3. 5 Ⓘ SLR
4. Able to discontinue immobilizer
5. If home discharge, has equip.
6. CPM ⇑ >90° and able until 90° passive ROM
7. SBA transfers
8. PROM 10°–80° POD #5, then increase as able

1. Rehabilitation of total knee postoperative day 5

2. F — Attend orthopedic rounds from 8:00–9:00 a.m.

3. Is patient going home today? — Yes → **4.** P

4. P
– give exercise handout to patient
– get walker or crutches for patient
– get portable raised toilet for patient
– obtain referral for outpatient or home physical therapy
– arrange for patient to take CPM home
– send knee immobilizer home with patient

5. Is patient to have physical therapy session now? — No / Yes

6. Check incision and swelling.

7. Is swelling minimal? — Yes / No

8. O — Discontinue Ace bandage.

9. E, J — CPM 0°–90° or more.

10. Rewrap knee with Ace bandage.

11. Have patient perform exercise TKR-POD 4.

12. Return patient to room after CPM session.

13. Can patient do 5 Ⓘ SLR's? — Yes / No

14. J — Discontinue immobilizer.

15. Notify nurse so bed can be changed.

16. Put knee immobilizer on.

17. Continue immobilizer use.

18. J — Sit EOB, AAROM measure with goniometer.

19. A — Ambulate 175 feet or more PWB with walker.

20. Is patient to ambulate now? — Yes / No

21. Return patient to supine position.

22. E, J — CPM on 0–90° measure range of motion with goniometer.

23. Was this a.m. Rx? — Yes / No

24. Chart; repeat process in p.m.

25. END

26. Contact nursing re CPM.

27. E — Chart

CLINICAL GUIDELINE DEVELOPMENT
Aspen Publishers, Inc.

ANNOTATIONS FOR TOTAL KNEE SURGERY

A. Preoperative Evaluation and Teaching

Usually, patients have preoperative examinations and hear explanations at Green Valley Physical Therapy as outpatients. Green Valley Physical Therapy will contact Evergreen Hospital therapy department regarding those who have undergone preoperative evaluations prior to surgery, and this information is posted on the bulletin board in the physical therapy department. As part of the preoperative evaluation, clinicians

- assess patient's functional ability to transfer and ambulate
- measure gross range of motion and strength in unaffected extremities
- measure range of motion (using goniometer) and grade strength in the surgical knee
- instruct the patient in TWB and PWB in walker and crutches
- instruct the patient in use of CPM, postoperative exercise program, and rehabilitation course

B. CPM

Call Sue Newman at Lyon's Medical Center Pharmacy at 555-3302 and order a CPM (refer to survival notebook for weekend staff). Give her the patient's name and room number and obtain a copy of the patient's billing information sheet (to be put on Lyon's clipboard in physical therapy department). Call Janet Night (ext 5498) and give her the patient's name, billing number, and room number. CPM will be delivered to the physical therapy department by Lyon's Pharmacy. Weekend staff will leave a message on the communication notebook for staff to call on Monday.

C. Fitting CPM

Use a measuring tape (or a gait belt) to measure the patient's surgical knee from the joint line to the bottom of the foot. Adjust the lower portion of the CPM to this length. Measure the medial thigh (from the joint line of the knee to just below the groin), and adjust the upper bracket of the CPM to this length. Apply a foot support pad, as well as lower leg and upper thigh pads, using Velcro straps. Ask a recovery room nurse to assist with applying the CPM by raising the surgical knee while the therapist slides CPM under the leg, making sure the joint line of the knee is aligned with the axis of the CPM. (Make sure the CPM is in extended position when applied.)

Plug in the CPM at the head of the bed so that the cord is out of the way. Put on the thigh and lower leg straps. Check the CPM range-of-motion setting and pre-set to 0 to 60 degrees with 1 minute per cycle speed setting (middle setting). (Patients who have spinal anesthesia usually do not get a return of sensation for 2 to 3 hours, so they can tolerate 0 to 60 degrees range of motion without warm-up.) Recheck the patient in his or her room within 2 hours. Record the CPM range of motion in the physical therapy flowchart.

D. Nursing Guidelines

Guidelines are stored in a file in the upper right cabinet directly behind the East wing unit secretary's desk. They are as follows:

- Maintain maximum elevation of knee and foot of bed for first 48 hours.
- After the first 48 hours, keep knee and foot of bed minimally gatched and elevated. Keep foot of bed straight. Maintain knee in extended position when not in CPM. *No pillows under knees.* Place pillow under heel of affected leg as much as tolerated.
- Rewrap Ace bandage on affected leg, foot to thigh, every shift. Wrapping may be discontinued on postoperative day 5 if swelling is under control.
- Knee immobilizer is to be worn during ambulation only. It will be discontinued when patient has good leg control (i.e., can perform five independent straight leg raises).

E. Provision of Information to Nursing Staff

Tell the patient's nurse what time the CPM is to come off (CPM should be on a minimum of 8 to 10 hours total). If the patient has been medicated and is still uncomfortable (and the therapist is gone for the day), have the nurse lower the range of motion by 5-degree increments until the patient is comfortable. (Do not go below 0 to 40 degrees, however.) Make sure the nurse knows how to remove the CPM and work the controls.

F. Orthopedic Rounds

Rounds usually start at 8:00 and end by 9:00 a.m. (Rounds usually begin in room 114 and end in room 106.) Bring copies of yesterday's flowsheets to rounds. Assist the orthopedic physician or physician assistant by giving information on the patient's ambulation distance, transfer ability, passive range of motion, and any other patient information. Notify the physician or physician assistant of any problems or questions with the patient's rehabilitation program.

G. Postoperative Day 1 Exercises

Have the patient perform 10 repetitions of each of the following exercises:

- ankle pumps
- hamstring sets
- quadricep sets
- gluteal sets
- upper extremity progressive resistive exercises

H. Jones Splint Removal and Dressing Change

Remove the soft Jones splint by unraveling the Ace bandage and cotton bandage, cutting the Kerlix bandaging, and carefully removing the sterile covering (wear protective gloves.) Have the nurse look at the wound before redressing. Check the wound for excessive drainage, poor closure, or possible infection. Clean with Betadine swabs over the incision site (especially over the staples), dress with Telfa pad, Kerlix bandage, and #6 tube gauze found in the clean supply room on the East wing on a cart. Reuse Ace bandage (if clean) to wrap the leg from foot to thigh (4-inch Ace bandage from foot to mid-lower leg, 6-inch Ace bandage from mid-lower leg to above the knee).

I. Transfer Technique

Supine to sitting. Lock the brakes of the bed or push the bed against the wall in preparation for transfer. Support the surgical leg, and have the patient assist as much as possible with the uninvolved leg and upper extremities. Provide as much assistance with the patient transfer as necessary (including a second person, if necessary). Help the patient to sit on the edge of the bed with the surgical leg touching the floor.

Sitting to standing. Place a transfer belt around the patient's trunk in a nonthreatening area. Make sure that IVs, catheter, and any other devices are clear and not obstructing movement. Have the pick-up walker in place. Make sure that the patient understands the weight-bearing status of the involved extremity. Have the patient use one hand to push off from the bed while holding onto the walker with the other hand, placing his or her full weight on the uninvolved lower extremity. Provide only as much assistance as necessary for a safe transfer. Communicate with the patient to determine his or her mental status and/or any complaints.

J. Measurement of Actual Range of Motion

Use goniometer to measure the actual range of motion. (Use greater trochanters and lateral malleoli as landmarks and lateral joint line for axis.)

CLINICAL GUIDELINE DEVELOPMENT
Aspen Publishers, Inc.

K. Use of Immobilizer

Measure mid-upper thigh circumference to determine size of knee immobilizer. Complete a requisition slip in Central Supply at the front desk. (Central Supply is down the hallway from the physical therapy department.) If none are available, leave a note at the front desk. Make sure the immobilizer is snug and will not slip off the patient during ambulation. Brace sizes are

1. small, 18 inches
2. medium, 20 inches
3. large, 22 inches
4. X-large, 24 inches
5. XX-large, 26 inches

L. Postoperative Day 2 Exercises

Have the patient do the postoperative day 1 exercises, but increase the number of repetitions to 15. (See G.) Begin active assistive straight leg raise, repeating the exercise 5 times. Place pillow under heel to increase extension two times per day for 15 minutes.

M. Postoperative Day 3 Exercises

Have patient increase isometric exercises to 20 repetitions. (See G and L.) Increase active assistive straight leg raise exercises to 10 repetitions.

N. Postoperative Day 4 Exercises

(See G, L, and M.) Begin attempts at independent straight leg raise. Begin active assisted range of motion at edge of bed and supine in bed.

O. Postoperative Day 5 Exercises

(See G, L, M, and N.) Continue with previous exercises. The patient should be able to do 5 repetitions of independent straight leg raise. Start short arc quadriceps exercise with blanket roll or pillow under thigh.

HOME EXERCISE PROGRAM

Provide patient with a home exercise program. Review exercises in order to make sure that the patient understands and can perform each exercise. Order any assistive devices and versamode (portable raised toilet) (if needed) from Lyon's Medical Center Pharmacy at 555-3302 (ask for Janet Night, if available). Determine whether the patient needs an outpatient referral or the services of a visiting nurse. The patient takes the CPM home for the first week to attain or maintain 0 to 90 degrees of motion.

Index